IN A NUTSHELL

IN A NUTSHELL

A quick guide to diet, health and fitness

Deryck Britton

ISBN: 9798594885547

Dedication

This book is dedicated to my wife, Deana

Table of Contents

Introduction

This book brings together many pieces of information on different aspects of general health, diet, and exercise. It contains 35 chapters which can be read in any order but maybe read from beginning to end. With each section containing compressed pieces of information from numerous sources, it is, hopefully, more easily digested than a bookcase full of books. In essence, it's a nutshell containing seeds of information. A reference section is at the back.

The idea for "In a Nut Shell" was put together after I passed a gym course called NABBA (National Armature Body Building Association). I'm not a body builder myself but I enjoyed going through the course. I do, however, enjoy general fitness: running, cycling, a bit gym work and when on holiday a swim.

At the time of finishing it, however, during the Covid19 lock down, I've more than put on a few pounds!

We sometimes set ourselves ambitions or goals for different reasons. Weather to run a half marathon or full marathon, to get fit for playing golf, or to cycle a few hundred miles. Or just to put one foot in front of the other. Or simply to keep fit. Some of us may be diabetic or have asthma, perhaps have a heart condition or through illness or injury have lost limbs. Confidence maybe lacking in some of us. And to gain confidence takes time. So by setting a goal we may gain confidence.

I've been lucky. I can run, swim or cycle even though I've got a chest defect called **pectus excavatum.**

My goal has all ways been simply to keep fit and hopefully help others. So I hope this little book may help.

Back in 2013 I took part in the Great North Run to raise money for the British Heart Foundation. My dad passed away in 2006 of heart problems. It took me seven years to gain confidence to run in that event.

So, that's the little intro bit over with.

Chapter 1

Vitamins

Vitamins are vital for the proper functioning of your body. There are 13 vitamins we need to get from food. They are: A, B complex (8 types), C, D, E, K. Vitamin B is actually a group of vitamins: B1, B2, B3, B5, B6, B7, B9, B12. The B group of vitamins have different names. They are:

- B1 thiamine
- B2 riboflavin
- B3 niacin
- B5 pantothenic acid
- B6 pyridoxine
- B7 biotin
- B9 folic acid
- B12 cobalamin

All types of B vitamin and vitamin C are water soluble which means they are not stored in the body, so we must make sure that we get these from our diet each day.

Vitamin A, D, E, K are fat soluble: your body can only absorb them with dentary fat intake.

Here is a quick overview of the roles these vitamins play in your body.

- Blood clotting: K
- Eye function: A
- Skin: A, B2, B5, B6, C
- Reproduction: A, B2
- Bones: A, C, D
- Blood formation: B6, B9, B12, C
- Blood cells: E

- Teeth: A, D, C
- Hormone formation: B5, B6
- Neuromuscular function: A, B1, B3, B5, B6, B12
- Cell membrane: E
- Energy release from food: B1, B2, B3, B5, B6, B7
- Antioxidant: A, B2, E
- Immune function: A
- ATP (adenosine triphosphate) formation. Every cell in your body produces ATP for energy.

What follows is look at the different types of vitamins, their role in our body, where we can find them in our foods and drinks, the recommended daily allowance (RDA); and important notes as to why we should not take in more than the RDA. Vitamins can be obtained naturally from a wide variety of foods.

Note: RDA is ether measured in milligrams mg (one thousandth of a gram); or in micrograms ug (one millionth of a gram).

Table showing the RDA for each vitamin

For men and women

Vitamin	Female	Male	Vitamin	Male	Male
A	700 ug	900 ug	B9	200 ug	200ug
B1	0.8 mg	1 mg	B12	1 ug	1 ug
B2	1.2 mg	1.6 mg	C	60 mg	60 mg
B3	1.4 mg	1.4 mg	D	5 ug	5 ug
B5	6 mg	6 mg	E	10 mg	10 mg
B6	2 mg	2 mg	K	65 mg	65 mg
B7	30 ug	30 ug			

Do not exceed the RDA as it may have a negative effect on the body

You should never overdose on vitamins or minerals. The following is a list of vitamins and minerals and their adverse effect when taken to excess.

- Vitamin A: can cause liver damage, hair loss, blurred vision and headaches. Pregnant women should avoid excessive amounts as this could cause birth defects.

- Vitamin B6: taking 200 times the recommended amount can cause numbness in the mouth and hands and difficulty in walking.

- Vitamin C: high doses can cause stomach ulcers and diarrhoea.

- Vitamin D: high doses can cause calcium deposits in the muscles, including the heart.

- B3: high amount (100 times RDA) could cause liver damage.

- B1: avoid high amounts as it could affect the absorption of other B vitamins.

Vitamin A (also called retinol)

- It is called retinol because it produces the pigments in the retina of the eye.

- Fat soluble vitamin.

- Essential for night vision, healthy skin, hair, bone formation, healthy cells; gene transcription, reproduction, embryonic development, fertility; boosts immunity, maintains healthy development and maintenance of teeth, soft tissue; needed for growth, and soft skeletal tissue.

- It is an antioxidant.

Deficiency symptoms:

- Night blindness.
- Low resistance to infection, and colds
- Dry skin.
- Mouth ulcers.

Sources:

Liver, cod liver oil, carrots, broccoli leaves, sweet potatoes, kale, butter, spinach, leafy vegetables, pumpkin, collard greens, cantaloupe, melon, eggs, apricots, paprika, mango, tomatoes, peas, winter squash, milk, cheddar cheese.

Note: Beta-carotene, a precursor of vitamin A, comes from highly coloured fruits and vegetables; and from leafy, green vegetables.

Vitamin B1 (Thiamine)

- It is essential for the continuous release of energy from carbohydrates.

- Needed for the transmission of electrical signals in the nerves and muscles.

- Important for the formation of red blood cells.

- Necessary for proper brain function.

- Needed for the digestive processes.

- Thiamine is found in both plants and animals.

- Needed for the formation of the energy carrier ATP in every cell in your body.

- Easily destroyed by heat.

Deficiency symptoms:

- Weakness and muscle pains,
- Water retention.

- Stomach pains.

- Poor concentration, nausea, beriberi, irritability.

Sources:

Yeast, oatmeal, grains, brown rice, wholemeal pasta, whole grain flour, asparagus, pork, kale, yeast extract, potatoes, oranges, pulses, cauliflower, peas, pulses, cured ham, liver (from beef, pork), eggs, fortified cereals.

Vitamin B2 (Riboflavin)

- Plays an important key role in energy metabolism food, especially fat and protein.

- Required for healthy skin and hair.

- Required for growth and reproduction.

- Helps to keep the skin healthy.

- Benefits vision.

- Helps to eliminate sore mouth, lips and tongue.

- Easily destroyed by sunlight.

Deficiency symptoms:

- Cracks in the skin at the corner of the mouth.

- Soreness of lips, mouth, and tongue.

- Anaemia.

- Cracked and dry lips (cheilosis).

- Scaling of the skin around the nose, mouth, scrotum, forehead, ears and scalp.

- Heightened sensitivity to light.

- Conjunctivitis and watering of the eyes.

Sources:

Liver, milk, cheese, yogurt, eggs, green vegetables, yeast extract, fortified cereals, kidney, fish, whole grains.

Vitamin B3 (Niacin)

- Essential for the nervous system.
- Needed for the production of sex hormones.
- It can be made in the body from the amino acid *tryptophan*.
- Essential for the release of energy from food.
- Helps to balance blood sugar and cholesterol levels.
- Needed for healthy skin and hair, digestive system.
- Required for proper brain function.
- Increases blood circulation and reduces blood pressure.

Deficiency symptoms:

- Leads to pellagra (inflation of the mouth).
- Poor memory.
- Anxiety, depression, fatigue.
- Eczema.
- Diarrhoea.

Sources:

Liver, heart, kidney, chicken, beef, tuna, salmon, eggs, avocados, dates, tomatoes, lead vegetables, broccoli, carrots, sweet potatoes, asparagus, nut, whole grain products, legumes, brewer's yeast.

Vitamin B5 (Pantothenic acid)

- Need for the conversion of food to energy.
- Essential for the conversion of choline to acetylcholine, a chemical messenger that carriers electrical signals between the nerves and muscles.
- Is easily destroyed by food processing.

Deficiency symptoms:

- Poor concentration.
- Anxiety.
- Fatigue.
- Tingling hands and feet.
- Muscle cramps.
- Headaches.
- Dizziness.

Sources:

Royal jelly, brewer's yeast, liver, kidney, nuts, whole grains, eggs, legumes, rice.

Vitamin B6 (Pyridoxine)

- Has to be present for B12 to be absorbed.
- Is a group of water soluble substances that work to together and are converted into the active form of pyridoxine in the body.
- Essential for the breakdown of foods.
- Needed for healthy brain function.

- Required for the breakdown of protein, fats, and carbohydrates.
- Needed for the synthesis of antibodies to support the immune system.
- It is used in the body as a catalyst in the reaction that involves amino acids.
- Blood cell formation.
- Keeps teeth and gums healthy.

Deficiency symptoms:

- Dry and cracking skin.
- Water retention.
- Anxiety, irritability, depression.
- Tingling hands, muscle cramps.
- Anaemia.

Sources:

Wheatgerm, bananas, yeast, chicken, soya beans, sunflower seeds, fish, Brussels sprouts, potatoes, wholemeal bread, leafy green vegetables, walnuts, baked beans, eggs.

Vitamin B7 (Biotin)

- Necessary for the release of energy from food, particularly form fats and carbohydrate.
- Correct muscle function.
- Required for health skin and hair.
- It is produced in small amounts by the bacteria in the intestines.

- Necessary for growth.
- Required for the production of fatty acids, antibodies, digestive enzymes.
- Needed for the metabolism of B3.

Deficiency symptoms:

- Anaemia, nausea, muscle pain.
- Depression, lethargy.
- Hair loss.
- Dermatitis.

Sources:

Meat, soya, fish, kidney, legumes, liver, wheat meal, bananas, peanut butter, poultry, egg yolk, oysters, beans, bread, nuts, legumes, brewer's yeast.

Note: egg white contains a chemical which strongly binds to biotin preventing it from being absorbed into the blood stream from the intestines.

Vitamin B9 (Folic acid)

- Works with many B vitamins.
- Works with B12 and vitamin C to help the body metabolise proteins; for the formation of amino acids; and the metabolism of sugars.
- Found in many foods; but is easily lost from the body.
- Required for cell division.
- Essential for the production of haem (the iron containing substance in haemoglobin) and for formation of red blood cells and oxygen transport.

- Highly important in the early stages of pregnancy.
- Required for the synthesis of DNA.
- Aids in digestion.

Deficiency symptoms:

- Anaemia.
- Cracked lips, sore tongue, cracking at the corners of the mouth.
- Depression.
- Lack of energy, fatigue.
- Poor appetite.
- Diarrhoea or constipation.
- Heartburn.
- Long term deficiency may cause osteoporosis, bowl cancer.

Sources:

Liver, leafy vegetables (spinach, broccoli, lettuce), dried beans and peas, fortified breakfast cereal, black eyed beans, sunflower seeds, peanuts, avocado, banana.

Vitamin B12 (Cobalamin)

- Maintains a health nervous system.
- Vital for the production of the myelin sheath – the covering that protects nerves and speeds up the passage of electrical signals along the length of the nerve.
- Needed for cell division.
- Required for production of red blood cells.

- Plays a key role in the normal functioning of the brain.

- Required for DNA synthesis.

- Needed for energy production.

- Fatty acid synthesis requires it.

- It is the largest and most structurally complex vitamin and can be produced industrially only through bacterial fermentation-synthesis.

Deficiency symptoms:

- Eczema or dermatitis.

- Poor memory.

- Anxiety and irritability.

- Sore and tender muscles.

- Pernicious anaemia – degeneration of the nerves cells.

Sources:

Liver, beef, eggs, cheese, fortified breakfast cereals, white fish, yeast extract, milk, chicken.

Vitamin C (Ascorbic acid)

- It is a strong antioxidant.

- Used to make collagen (the protein that makes skin, bones and joints strong).

- Needed for healthy teeth.

- Necessary for the absorption of iron.

- Required for the growth and repair of tissue.

- Maintains a healthy immune system.

Deficiency symptoms:

- Bleeding gums.
- Aches and pains.
- Red pimples on the skin; skin bruises easily.
- Poor wound healing, scurvy, nosebleeds.

Sources:

Citrus fruits, vegetables, liver, potatoes.

Vitamin D (Calciferol)

- The body produces vitamin D when exposed to sunlight.
- Vital for the absorption of the minerals calcium and phosphorus which is vital for the development and strength of healthy bones and teeth, especially during childhood.
- Needed for the proper functioning of the heart.

Deficiency symptoms:

- Backache, tooth decay.
- Twisted limbs in children, rickets.
- Brittle and painful bones.

Sources:

Cod liver oil, herrings, mackerel, sardines, salmon, margarine, tuna, and cheddar cheese.

Vitamin E (Tocophrol)

- It is an antioxidant.
- Helps to improve the activity of vitamin A.

- Helps in the formation of red blood cells.
- Necessary for muscle function.
- It is a fat soluble vitamin retained in the body for a short time, so needs to be re replaced regularly.
- Needed for a healthy heart, blood supply and blood formation.
- Reduces abnormal blood clotting.
- Protects the cell walls, tissues from damage by oxidation; helps to fight free radicals – which causes ageing – and so help the skin to keep looking young.

Deficiency symptoms:

- Skin easily bruised.
- Slow wound healing.
- Exhaustion after exercise.
- Varicose veins.
- Dietary intake may not be enough.

Sources:

Wheat germ oil, sunflower oil, sunflower seeds, nuts, green leafy vegetables, wheat germ, almonds, peanut butter, asparagus, avocado, eggs.

Vitamin K

- Necessary for the blood to coagulate; and for bleeding to stop.
- Required for proper wound healing.
- Bacteria in the human colon synthesizes a significant amount of vitamin K.

Deficiency symptoms:

- Excessive bleeding after injury.
- Spontaneous bleeding.

Sources:

Green leafy vegetables e.g. spinach, broccoli, lettuce, cabbage, sprouts, cauliflower; cow's milk, banana, avocado, kiwi, grapes, fortified breakfast cereals.

Chapter 2
Minerals

Your body requires a number of important minerals in order for it function properly. Vitamins and minerals are called micronutrients (or trace elements). Your body needs theses trace elements in varying amounts which can normally be obtained from a diet which contains a wide range of foods stuffs. Most are vital; and some are trace elements. Some are electrolytes.

An **electrolyte** is a mineral that dissolves in water and carries an electric charge. The minerals potassium, Sodium and chloride are electrolytes, and because they dissolve in water they are found everywhere in the body. They are vital for every cell of the body. Calcium and magnesium are also electrolytes.

Drinking too much water without replacing electrolytes could cause neurological problems or death.

All living cells on earth require potassium, sodium and chloride which means that there are plenty of those minerals in natural food; but not so in processed food; and which have a high sodium content.

Just a brief note on chloride:

In your body the mineral chlorine takes the form of chloride. It is important in maintain water balance; and is an essential component of gastric juice (hydrochloric acid). We get our main supply of chlorine from salt (sodium chloride).

Dietary deficiency of chlorine is rare. But can occurs if you have excessive loss from your body. This can result from pronged vomiting, diarrhoea, or sweating.

The table on the next page show the minerals with their related atomic symbol. A Balanced diet should provide the minerals that your body requires each day.

- Calcium   Ca
- Copper   Cu
- Iodine   I
- Iron   Fe
- Magnesium   Mg
- Phosphorus   P
- Potassium   K
- Sodium   Na
- Zinc   Zn

Calcium

- Nearly all of your intake of calcium goes straight to the bones and teeth. Only a small amount is left to circulate around the body.

- Needed for muscle contraction.

- Required for the blood to clot.

- Need for nerve impulses.

- Helps to maintain your immune system.

- Keeps your heartbeat regular, maintains blood pressure.

- For your body to absorb calcium, vitamin D has to be present. (Your body naturally produces vitamin D in sunlight.)

- Your body uses calcium every day and must be replaced in the diet each day.

- If dietary intake is low the body takes calcium from bones and teeth.

Deficiency symptoms:

- Sleeplessness.
- Muscle cramps or twitching.
- Arthritis or other joint pains.
- High blood pressure.
- Tooth decay.

Note: calcium works with phosphate. High intake of phosphate will restrict the intake of calcium. Phosphorus is another very important mineral that your body needs.

RDA: 800 mg – 1000 mg

Sources:

Milk, cheddar cheese, sardines, tofu, dried egg, watercress, yogurt, cabbage, eggs, canned fish, white flour, bread, green leafy vegetables.

Copper

- Required for blood cell formation and function.
- Needed for bone formation.
- Required for proper heart functioning.
- The body cannot synthesise copper and must be obtained from diet.
- Stored in the liver. Normal levels are maintained by the body given a balanced diet.
- Combines with certain proteins to produce enzymes that help a number of body functions. Some help provide energy required by biochemical reactions.
- Required for the formation and repair of collagen and elastin in connective tissue.

- Too much copper intake or too little may result in tissue injury and disease.

Deficiency symptom: may cause anaemia.

RDA: 1.2 mg/day

Sources:

Green vegetables, fish and liver, dried fruit.

Iodine

- Essential for the production of thyroid hormones, which control your metabolic rate and your energy levels. A high metabolic rate help you to burn fat.
- Regulates growth.
- Vital for a child's physical and mental development. In the early years.
- Is a component of almost every living plant and animal.
- High levels can be toxic.

Deficiency symptoms

- Increased risk of retarded brain development.
- Mental slowness, poor concentration and memory problems.
- High cholesterol, weight gain.
- Lethargy, fatigue, depression.
- Swelling of the thyroid gland (goitre).
- Cold hands and feet.

RDA: 140 ug

Sources:

Kelp, haddock, cod, condensed milk, eggs, mayonnaise, cheddar cheese, malt bread, naan bread.

Iron

- Used in the production of haemoglobin and myoglobin. Myoglobin is an iron and oxygen binding protein found in the muscle tissue of vertebrates. It is related to haemoglobin, which is the iron and oxygen binding protein in the blood.

- Used to transport oxygen to all parts of the body and removal of waste.

- Avoid drinking tea with, or just before, a meal as this can interfere with iron absorption.

- Vitamin C helps with the absorption of iron.

- Too much iron intake could lead to the production of free-radicals. These cause damage to every cell in the body, which accelerate the ageing process.

- Strengthens the immune system.

- Promotes healthy growth and development.

Deficiency symptoms:

- Pail skin, itchiness.

- White or brittle nails.

- Tiredness, frequent illnesses, fatigue, weakness, shortness of breath, insomnia, headache.

- Loss of appetite.

- Impaired concentration.

RDA: 14 mg

Sources:

Fortified breakfast cereals, liver, dried fruit, sardines, canned tuna, parsley, watercress, flour, eggs, red meat, spinach, and tofu.

Magnesium

- Is essential for every biochemical process in the body. Examples ATP, DNA, enzyme syntheses.

- Relaxes muscles after contraction.

- Needed for turning protein, carbohydrates, fats into energy.

- Critical for muscles and nerves.

- Keeps bones and teeth strong. About 65% of magnesium is found in the bones, 25% in the muscles with the remainder in cells, soft tissue, fluids etc.

- Absorption is less efficient in the presence of alcohol, calcium, protein, phosphates and fats.

- Absorption is more efficient when vitamin D is present.

- Helps to fight depression.

- Plays a part in the hormone insulin.

- Crucial for the synthesis of genetic material.

- Unabsorbed magnesium goes straight through your body; absorbed magnesium, is lost through sweat and urine. Loss through urine is regulated by the kidneys.

RDA: 300 mg

Deficiency symptoms:

Depression, fits, tiredness, irritability, stress, irregular heartbeat, cramp or twitching muscles, sleeplessness.

Sources:

Potatoes, bananas, eggs, milk, nuts, seafood, tomatoes, brown sugar, cereals, hot coca, green peas, cheddar cheese, spinach. Small amount in orange juice.

Phosphorus

- Essential for healthy bones and teeth.
- Major constituent of all cells.
- Required for the formation of DNA and ATP.
- Vitamin D is needed for the body to absorb phosphorus.
- Every cell has a boundary that contains phosphorus: the phospholipid layer.

Deficiency symptoms:

- Weight loss, feeling weak, fatigue and stress, tremors.
- Growth and tooth problems, rickets.
- Skin sensitivity.
- Irregular breathing.
- Muscle and neurological dysfunction.

Sources:

Oats, whole wheat, bran, milk, cottage cheese, beans, , nuts, seeds, chicken, turkey, egg yolk, fish, crab, shrimp, clams, , rice, bread, yeast, pluses.

Potassium

- Is an electrolyte.

- Essential for nerve, heart and muscle functions.

- A normal balance of potassium to sodium in the ratio 2:1 should be maintained. Which is twice as much potassium as sodium in the body.

- High blood pressure is a result of too much sodium and not enough potassium.

Deficiency symptoms:

- Weakness, muscle cramps.

- Mental confusion.

- In extreme cases heart failure.

RDA: 3500 mg

Sources:

Banana, avocado, beef, black beans, lentils, milk, orange, carrot, chicken, sweat potatoes, spinach, cantaloupe, winter squash, tomatoes, wheat germ, kiwi, strawberries, kidney beans, watermelon.

Sodium

- Is an electrolyte.
- Regulates blood volume, blood pressure and pH.
- Regulates water balance in the body.
- Essential for muscle, nerve and heart function.
- There is a potassium/sodium balance which is 2:1 that is twice as much potassium to sodium.
- High levels of sodium in the diet causes high blood pressure.

Deficiency symptoms:

Electrolyte unbalance, muscles cramps, dizziness. Could cause heart failure.

RDA: 1600 mg

Sources:

Main source in the diet is from salt (sodium chloride).

Zinc

- Vital for growth and repair.
- Involved with enzyme activity.
- Required for taste perception.
- Healthy skin and hair.
- Required for fertility in both men and women.
- It fuels everything from manufacturing DNA, wound healing, maintaining a strong immune system, to fighting colds, flu and other infections.

- The human body does not produce zinc, so it must be obtained from the diet.

Deficiency symptoms:

- May cause delayed puberty and retarded growth.
- Frequent infections.
- Poor wound healing.
- Loss of sense of taste or smell.
- Eczema, acne or psoriasis.
- White flecks in the fingernails, slow nail or hair growth.
- Poor appetite.

RDA: 150 mg

Sources:

Beef, brown rice, cheddar cheese, chicken, crab, eggs, fortified cereals, ham, lamb, liver, milk, oysters, pork, pulses, seafood, turkey, wheat germ, white rice.

Chapter 3

Carbohydrates at a glance

There are two types of carbohydrates: simple (sugars); and complex (starches and fibres). All carbohydrates are broken down into **glucose** to produce energy. Glucose found in foods is commonly called **grape sugar**; and in the human body is called **blood sugar**. Once the carbohydrate has been broken down by the digestive system, **insulin** is released by the **pancreas** to transport the glucose through the bloodstream to sites where they are needed to provide energy, or to be stored as **glycogen** in the liver and muscles, which can be used later if needed. But only a small amount can be stored this way; any glycogen that cannot be stored in the liver and muscles is stored as fat in fat cells.

Complex carbohydrates are so named because they are comprised of very complicated structures. These are the carbs that are most often referred to as starch and fibre. They are more difficult for the body to break down rapidly, which ensures a longer, more sustained supply of energy to the body.

These are broken down into glucose more slowly than simple carbs. Most natural complex carbohydrate sources also provide vitamins and minerals necessary for the efficient conversion to ATP (see chapter 22). If these vitamins and minerals are not present some of the carbs may be turned into fat and stored.

Glucose is used as rapidly as it is produced. It enables the brain, nervous system, muscles and other organs to function.

Some natural complex carbohydrates:

Wholegrain bread, oats, brown rice, bran, barley, maze, buckwheat, cornmeal, oatmeal, pasta, macaroni, potatoes, root vegetables, pitta bread, bagel, wholegrain cereals, porridge oats, all bran, Weetabix, shredded wheat, ryvita, muesli.

Simple carbohydrates have one or two sugar units. These include **monosaccharides** (one sugar): **glucose** (dextrose), **fructose** (fruit sugar), and **galactose**. And the **disaccharides** (2 sugar units): **sucrose** (table sugar), which comprises a glucose and a fructose molecule joined together; (milk sugar).

Some simple carbohydrate fruits:

Apple, blackcurrants, kiwi, plum, pear, peach, raspberries, cherries.

Simple carbohydrates are broken down by the body very quickly to produce energy. They give a quick but short release of energy.

In a normal meal the percentage of carbohydrate should be about 60% of the total calorie intake.

As an example a person whose daily calorie intake is 2500 Kcal would expect their carbohydrate intake to be:

2500 x 0.6 = 1500 Kcal (0.6 is 60%).

And in terms of grams:

1500 / 3.75 (as 1 gram of carbohydrate provides 3 ¾ Kcal).

Which is 400 grams of carbs daily intake split between different meals of the day.

Chapter 4

Protein

You may have thought that protein is only needed to make your muscles grow. Not so. Every cell in your body requires protein: skin, hair, nails, tendons, internal organs, eyes. Well you get drift. Proteins are essential nutrient for the human body._They are one of the building blocks of your body. It can, in times of need, also serve as a fuel source. As fuel, protein contains 4 kcal per gram, a bit more than carbohydrates, which have 3.75 kcal per gram and unlike lipids (fats), which contain 9 kcal per gram.

The normal percentage of protein to body weight is about 20%. But this of cause can vary greatly. Body builders would have a much higher percentage and aim to reduce fat.

Protein is made from building blocks called amino acids. There are 20 different types of amino acids.

- Refer to the section on amino acids for more information.

What does protein do?

Protein is needed to regulate correct fluid balance in the tissues, to regulate metabolic pathways, transporting products into and out of cells. For caring oxygen around the body. Regulates blood clotting. Gives structure and strength to cells. Allows you to move. Needed to all the body's enzymes and to make various hormones like:

- Adrenaline: increases the rate of blood circulation, breathing and regulates carbohydrate metabolism.

- Insulin: lowers the blood sugar (glucose) levels in the blood.

Daily protein intake.

How much protein you can digest at one mealtime depends on you gender, muscle mass and how hard you train. Also if you increase your protein intake over time your body produces more enzymes to absorb the protein. Your body can only absorb 25-35g of protein at any one time. If a meal contains more than this the excess is excreted in your urine while extra calories will be laid down as fat. You need more daily protein during adolescence and if you wish to increase muscle mass.

In a normal meal the percentage of protein should be about 15% of the total calorie intake. And for the overall daily calories intake again 15%. Some meals might only contain 8% or less, and others might contain 20%. But during the course of the day this should average out.

So for example:

If your daily calorie intake was 2500 Kcal per day, your daily protein intake would be 15% of this.

A way to work this out is to times 2500 by 0.15 giving 2500 x 0.15 = 375 Kcal in total per day (0.15 is 15%)

Now as each gram of protein contains 4 Kcal we need to divide this by 4 to give the amount of grams of protein per day:

375 /4 = 93.75 or about 94 grams of protein per day.

You can only digest a small amount of protein at a time. If you ingest more protein than can be digested it is turned into fat.

Chapter 5

Fats and cholesterol

There are several types of fat: some our bodies need to function – essential fats; and others that are best avoid (saturated fat).

Saturated fats (the bad fats).

This type of fat is found in meat, fatty sausages, pastries, cakes, biscuits, chocolate, lard, butter, coconut and palm oil. Having too much saturated fat in the diet can increase the total amount of cholesterol in the blood. This in turn increases the risk of developing heart disease. Saturated fats increase both good and bad cholesterol.

Unsaturated fats, or the good fats.

Unsaturated fats don't raise cholesterol in the same way that saturated fats do. There are two types of unsaturated fats: Polyunsaturated and monounsaturated.

Polyunsaturated fats.

This type of fat lowers the total cholesterol (that is both good and bad) in the blood when substituted for saturated fat. This decreases the risk of developing heart disease.

Polyunsaturated fat can be found in vegetable oil, sunflower oil, oily fish (omega 3 fatty acids).

Mono unsaturated fats.

Monounsaturated fats are the most beneficial because they lower bad cholesterol without adversely affecting the good cholesterol (which is cardio protective) Examples of monounsaturated fats include olive oil, ground nut oil, rapeseed oil, nuts.

Omega 3 fatty acid is an essential fatty acid

Omega 3 fatty acids have been shown to protect against coronary heart disease – helps to keep your heart healthy. It supports the normal development of the brain, eyes, and nerves. Oily fish is the best source: mackerel, herring, salmon, sardines, trout, pilchards, kipper, eel, whitebait, and fresh tuna.

Omega 6 is also an essential fatty acid.

Omega 6 fatty acid can be found in corn, sunflower oil, margarine, soya bean oil, cotton seed oil, mayonnaise.

The human body cannot synthesize omega 3 or 6 fatty acid from scratch; but both are essential for normal body functions. However, too much omega 6 is harmful. The current recommended ratio of omega 6 to 3 is 4-5 to 1. Western diets very from 10 to 1 to as high as 30 to1.

Trans fats

Trans fats cannot be broken down in the body. They have the same effect as saturated fats. They are found in biscuits, cakes, fast foods, pastry, palm oil and some margarines. They are formed when liquid vegetable oils are turned into solid fats through the process of hydrogenation.

What is cholesterol?

Cholesterol is a fat produced in the liver and is essential for correct body functioning. Cell walls need cholesterol to remain healthy. Some hormone and digestive juices also need cholesterol. We all produce cholesterol from the fats we eat, but some people produce more than others and this is where raised cholesterol problems start. Measuring good and bad cholesterol is a way to determine if you are using and cleaning away excess cholesterol efficiently.

A brief note on good and bad cholesterol.

Fats are insoluble in water but need to be transported in the blood; this is achieved by *lipoproteins*. High density lipoproteins (HDL) transports excess cholesterol from tissues and other lipoproteins back to the liver. It reduces the level of fat in the blood and as a result plays a part in protecting the heart against atherosclerosis. HDL is said to be good cholesterol.

Low density lipoproteins (LDL) are rich in cholesterol and they act as an external source of cholesterol for cells. LDL is associated with higher risk of coronary heart disease; and is said to be bad cholesterol.

Recommended Daily fat intake.

As an example for daily fat intake, we will take an individual whose daily calorie intake is 2500 Kcal. We will take a daily fat intake of 25% of the total calorie intake. This is just a rough guide.

25% of 2500 is 625 Kcal.

This is total amount of daily calories that should come from fat. Now because there are 9 calories per 1 gram of fat we need to find the amount of fat in terms of grams. That is 69 grams to the nearest gram. So the maximum intake of fat for the day would be 69 grams. But as we have seen there are different types of fat.

A brief note on the condition **atherosclerosis**. (Arteriosclerotic Vascular Disease.) This is a condition in which the arterial walls thicken due to fatty deposits and cholesterol. These substances get into the lining of the arteries at sites which have microscopic damage, and there accumulate to form athermanous plaque, on top of which is a fibrous cap. The plaque narrows the space (lumen) within the arteries causing disturbances in the blood flow, which may cause eddies and these could lead to clots forming.

Chapter 6
Fibre in thy diet

Fibre in your diet is very important for a number of reasons:

- It lowers blood cholesterol.

- Helps to control blood sugar levels and therefore controls appetite.

- Helps the digestive system to process food and absorb nutrients.

- Helps to prevent heart disease.

- Helps to prevent weight gain.

- Keeps your intestines healthy.

Fibre is found in plant based foods.

There are two types of fibre:

- Soluble.

- Insoluble.

Soluble fibre

This dissolves in the water in your digestive system. The level of cholesterol in your blood may be reduced by the consumption of soluble fibre. It is found such as rye, oats, barley, fruit (such as bananas, apples), root vegetables (such as carrots, potatoes).

Insoluble fibre

This passes through your gut without being dissolved and helps food move through your gut more easily. In essence keeps your bowels healthy. It is found in foods such as bran, wholemeal bread, cereals, nuts and seeds (but not golden linseeds).

- A note of caution to this tale: too much fibre might give you a bit of wind!

Chapter 7

Daily water requirements

Have you ever stopped what you're doing and asked the question, "Why do we need water?"

- Well, Water makes up 50 to 70 per cent of an adult's total body weight and, without regular top-ups, our body's survival time is limited to a matter of days.
- Water's essential for the body's growth and maintenance, as it's involved in a number of processes. For example, it helps get rid of waste and regulates temperature, and it provides a medium for biological reactions to occur in the body.
- Water's lost from the body through urine, sweat and every time we breathe out; and it must be replaced frequently through diet.
- If you don't consume enough you can become dehydrated, causing symptoms such as headaches, tiredness and loss of concentration. Chronic dehydration can contribute to a number of health problems such as constipation and kidney stones.

How much water do we need?

Well, drinking pure water is essential as it flushes out toxins from the body; but the body may get it's **fluids** from these sources:

- Drinks, either plain water or as part of other beverages including tea, coffee and squash.

- Solid foods, especially fruit and vegetables (even foods such as bread and cheese provide small amounts of fluid).
- As a by-product of chemical reactions within the body.
- Most healthy adults need between one and a half to three litres a day, so aim to drink six to eight medium glasses of fluid daily. Beverages such as tea, coffee and fruit juices count towards fluid intake, and may bring with them other nutrients or benefits.
- You may require more fluid if you're very physically active or during periods of hot weather.
- You can judge whether you're drinking enough water by the colour of your urine. If it's a pale straw colour then your fluid intake is probably fine. If your urine is dark yellow, you probably need to drink more.
- Don't drink too much pure water while exercising as this could flush out your electrolytes to a very low level, which in extreme cases may cause death. Levels of potassium and sodium must be maintained. Some sports drinks contain electrolytes.

How to maintain fluid levels

- Start as you mean to go on, with a glass of water when you wake.
- Find time to make yourself regular drinks during the day - don't forget that tea, coffee and juices can count. Just watch out for the amount of sugar consumed in some soft drinks.
- Keep a bottle of water with you when travelling or exercising.
- Get into the habit of having a glass of water with every meal.
- The sensation of thirst is not triggered until you're already dehydrated, so it's important to drink before you get thirsty.

- Increase your intake of fresh fruit and vegetables, as they have a high water content and they contain vitamins and minerals.

Bottled water

- In some parts of the world like the U.K you can drink water straight from the tap; and in other places you have to buy bottled water to drink: an example would be Spain.

- There are two types: spring water and mineral water.

- Spring water is collected directly from the spring where it rises from the ground, and must be bottled at the source. UK sources of spring water must meet certain hygiene standards, and may be further treated so they meet pollution regulations.

- Mineral water emerges from under the ground, then flows over rocks before it's collected, resulting in a higher content of various minerals. Unlike spring water, it can't be treated except to remove grit and dirt. Different brands of spring and mineral waters have differing amounts of minerals depending on their source.

Chapter 8
Amino acids
The Essential and None Essential

Firstly, amino acids are the building block of proteins in your body. These amino acids are combined in different ways to produce the many types of protein and enzymes that your body uses. Protein is needed for repair and growth of everything from skin, internal organs, hair and nails. Protein accounts for about 20% of your total body weight.

There are a total of 20 of these amino acids, split into two groups. One group of eight are essential because our bodies cannot produce them and have to be in our diet. They are required for our bodies to be healthy and function properly. The other twelve are none essential ones that can be produced in your bodies from other amino acids, carbohydrate and nitrogen if they are lacking in your diet.

Below is a table listing the names of the essential and none essential amino acids.

Essential (EAA)	None essential (NEAA)
Isoleucine	Alanine
Leucine	Arginine
Lysine	Asparagine
Methionine	Aspartic acid
Phenylalanine	Cysteine
Threonine	Glutamic acid
Tryptophan	Glutamine

Valine

Glycine

Histidine

Proline

Serine

Tyrosine

The table below lists where the essential amino acids may be found.

Essential amino acid (EAA)	Sources (not exhaustive)
Isoleucine	Eggs, soy protein, seaweed, turkey, chicken, lamb, cheese and fish.
Leucine (L-Leucine is classed as a flavour enhancer E641)	Soy protein concentrate, peanuts, wheat germ, almonds, oats, beans, lentils, chickpea, corn (yellow), rice (brown).
Lysine	Red meat, eggs, watercress, soy bean, lentil, most beans, asparagus pea, spinach, buckwheat.
Methionine	Sesame seeds, Brazil nuts, soy protein concentrate, wheat germ, oats, peanuts, chickpea, corn (yellow), almonds, beans, lentils, rice (brown).

Phenylalanine	Egg white dried, soy protein isolate, de fatted peanut flour, de fatted soy flour, dried white fish, tofu, soy beans, dried parsley, butter nuts.
Phenylalanine	Edam cheese, cheddar cheese, kidney beans, dry whole milk with added vitamin D, Colby cheese, Cheshire cheese, peanut butter.
Threonine	Cottage cheese, poultry, fish, meat, lentils, sesame seeds.
Typtophan	Chocolate, oats, dried date, milk, yoghurt, cottage, cheese, red meat, eggs, fish, poultry, sesame seeds, chick peas, sunflower seeds, pumpkin seeds, peanuts
Valine	Most cheeses, egg white, milk dry none fat, game, lamb, veal, fish: cod, pike, tuna, haddock, perch, Pollock, grouper, pout, sunflower seeds, sesame seeds, soy protein isolate, soy britein concentrate, soy sauce made from soy, soy flower, tofu, watercress.

By eating a wide and varied selection of foods each week you should be able to supply your body with all the essential amino acids that it needs.

Branch chain amino acids (BCAA) contain three essential amino acids (EAA): valine, leucine and isoleucine. They make one third of muscle protein and are vital for glutamine and alanine, which are used during intensive aerobic exercise, like running. They can also be used directly by the muscles when glycogen, which is fuel for muscles, is depleted.

Chapter 9
Free radicals and antioxidants

Just what are free radical? In essence free radicals in our body contribute to cell damage, which over the years is what we see as ageing and age related medical conditions.

The human body is composed of many different types of cells. Cells are composed of many different types of molecules. Molecules consist of one or more atoms of one or more elements joined by chemical bonds.

Free radicals brake these bonds because they themselves are electrically unstable.

The most important structural feature of an atom for determining its chemical behaviour is the number of electrons in its outer shell. A substance that has a full outer shell tends not to enter in chemical reactions (an inert substance). Because atoms seek to reach a state of maximum stability, an atom will try to fill its outer shell by:

1. Gaining or losing electrons to either fill or empty its outer shell.

2. Sharing its electrons by bonding together with other atoms in order to complete its outer shell.

Atoms often complete their outer shells by sharing electrons with other atoms. By sharing electrons, the atoms are bound together and satisfy the conditions of maximum stability for the molecule.

How free radicals are formed?

Normally, bonds don't split in a way that leaves a molecule with an odd, unpaired electron. But when weak bonds split, free radicals are formed. Free radicals are very unstable and react quickly with other compounds, trying to capture the needed electron to gain stability. Generally, free radicals attack the nearest stable molecule, "stealing" its electron. When the "attacked" molecule loses its electron, it becomes a free radical itself, beginning a chain reaction. Once the process is started, it can cascade, finally resulting in the disruption of a living cell.

Some free radicals arise normally during metabolism. Sometimes the body's immune system purposefully create them to neutralize viruses and bacteria. However, environmental factors such as pollution, radiation, sun light, cigarette smoke and herbicides can also spawn free radicals.

Antioxidants

The vitamins C and E are called antioxidants. These are thought to protect the body against the destructive effects of free radicals. Antioxidants neutralize free radicals by donating one of their own electrons, ending the electron "stealing" reaction. The antioxidant nutrients themselves don't become free radicals by donating an electron because they are stable in either form. They act as scavengers, helping to prevent cell and tissue damage that could lead to cellular damage and disease.

- Vitamin E: the most abundant fat-soluble antioxidant in the body and one of the most efficient chain-breaking antioxidants available. Primary defender against oxidation.

- Vitamin C: the most abundant water-soluble antioxidant in the body. Acts primarily in cellular fluid. Of particular note in combating free-radical formation caused by pollution and cigarette smoke. Also helps return vitamin E to its active form.

44

Chapter 10

Daily calorie intake verses daily calorie usage and a bit on diets

Your body needs energy to function. Every activity requires your body to use energy. Just being sat down reading the newspaper requires energy: reading, thinking, holding the paper, the beating of your heart, movement of the chest, being sat straight, to the functioning of the internal organs, all requires energy. Energy that you gain from food and drink – this is what we know as calories. But if you take in too much energy, too many calories – be it in the form of carbohydrates, protein, alcohol or fat – any that you don't use gets turned into fat. That's' right – it's not just fat, in your diet that gets to sit around our middle: energy that your body doesn't use gets stored in fat cells around your body. Daily calorie intake can also called daily energy requirements.

These fat cells are produced when you are baby and stay with you for the rest of your life. These fat cells may be produced anywhere; but mainly around the tummy.

Your body is totally reliant on what you eat. There is a very simple rule about the amount of calories you need to consume in one day: to maintain weight only take enough calories that you need. Too few and you will lose weight; too many and you will gain weight. And don't forget ... you are what you eat!

We are all different in size and build; and we all have different activities in our daily life. Because of this your daily calorie requirements vary to what your body needs, and to what we as individuals have set as goals for ourselves. You might be wanting to gain muscle mass, to prepare yourself for a marathon, to lose a bit of weight and be toned up, or to strengthen your core and back muscles.

The table below shows how much energy 1 gram of protein, carbohydrate, fat and alcohol provides.

1 gram of protein provides	4 kcal
1 gram of carbohydrate provides	3.75 kcal
1 gram of fat (lipids) provides	9 kcal
1 gram of alcohol provides	7 kcal

Our bodies need a certain percentage of carbohydrate to protein to fat (by the way these are called macronutrients) together with vitamins and minerals (the micronutrients) and water to function properly.

The ratio in a normal meal is:

Macronutrient Breakdown

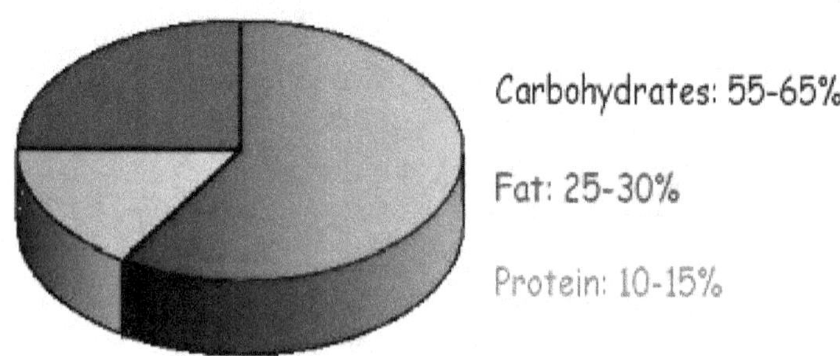

This ratio changes somewhat if we wish to exercise to gain muscle mass: carbohydrate 60%, fat 10% max, and protein 30%.

For example diets, refer to separate section called **A selection of diet plans.**

Except for the special diets, exercise plays an important part in achieving your goal: you won't win Mr Universe without hard work in gym and a diet to build muscle while reducing fat – which include cardiovascular work; or run a marathon without a combination of carbs, protein and fat combined with endurance running and mild resistance training to maintain muscle mass, as your body will breakdown muscle for energy use (this is because it takes longer to turn fat back into usable energy than it takes to turn muscle into usable energy). Also muscle stores glycogen which the body uses for energy.

So a very important note to remember here is: to burn of fat you need cardiovascular work and you need to work your muscles, to stop them being broken down for quick fuel.

Metabolism

Metabolism is term given to the sum all biochemical processes that occur in your body. The liver, brain, heart, kidneys, skeletal muscles and other organs account for about 70% of the total energy expenditure; a further 20% from our physical activity; and the last 10% comes from digestion of food and thermogenesis (the process of heat production in organisms).

Some people have a fast metabolism. They have a very good apatite but gain little weight, even without doing huge amounts of physical activity. Some have a slow metabolism, eat a normal amount of food but gain weight easily. They might exercise to try to reduce their weight but find it hard. And some people have a metabolism that is just right, who find it easy to keep their weight to an ideal level. The thyroid gland controls metabolism. This is done by secreting hormones. It is found in the throat under the larynx.

There are 2 types of metabolic rate:

- **Basal metabolic rate** (BMR) is the rate at which the body expends energy at total rest. That is not digesting food (approximately 12 hours after consuming food); and that the person's sympathetic nervous system is not stimulated: that is to say sleeping. It accounts for more than two-thirds of total energy expenditure.

- **Resting metabolic rate** is the rate at which the body burns calories at rest but not sleeping.

Once we know a person's BMR we can approximately work out the individual's daily calorie intake to maintain that person's weight. From this we can then estimate what the person's daily calorie intake would be to maintain weight, to lose weight, to gain weight, or calorie intake for sport, etc.

To estimate a person's BMR we can use the formula:

(Body weight in kg) x 24 for men;

(Body weight in kg x 0.9) x 24 for women.

And to estimate a person's daily energy requirements we can use the formula:

Kcal (per day) = BMR x 1.6.

As an example a man who weighs 70kg would have an approximate BMR of:

- 70*24 = 1680 for his BMR.
- So daily calorie intake is 1680 * 1.6 gives 2688 Kcal.

However, remember that this is just an estimate because not everyone has the same metabolism: the above number (2688

Kcal) maybe too high for someone who weighs 70kg; and maybe too low for somebody else who also weighs 70kg; and factors like how physical their job might be, what activities they might do each day.

A small note:

- A safe daily increase in calorie requirement to gain weight would be 10%. But again this has to be done with the right balance of protein to carbohydrate to fat. A meal replacement drink is ideal for those who are very active, eat very well but still find it hard to gain weight. As an example I was nine and a half stone at 20, and only about ten and a half stone when I got married at 27. During those years I tried meal replacement drinks which helped me to gain a little weight.

- Similarly to lose weight a decrease of 10% of daily calorie intake should not be exceeded; and should be combined with resistance and cardiovascular training.

Chapter 11
Digestion

Digestion! It's just one word, but a lot goes on from when you eat until your body can make use of that meal. So, read on and let's start the journey!

Food is initially broken down for digestion by a combination of chewing and grinding by the teeth and by a small amount of enzymes produced by three pairs of salivary glands: the **parotids** (located in front of and just below each ear), the **submaxillary gland** (located on the inner sides of the lower jaw bone), and the **sublingual glands** (in the floor of the mouth, below the tongue).

Saliva is made up of 99.5% water, it also contains solutes like **amylase**, an enzyme that begins the breakdown of salts and starches. Saliva lubricates food and makes chewing and swallowing easer. It also keeps the mouth moist between periods of eating.

Once food has been chewed and lubricated, the ball of food – called a **bolus** – is pushed to the back of the mouth by the tongue. Automatic reflexes push the bolus down the **pharynx**, at the same time moves the **epiglottis** over the **trachea** to prevent bolus from 'going down the wrong way'. From the pharynx the bolus travels down the **oesophagus** to the stomach.

The stomach is dotted with deep pits from which are secreted various substances. **Hydrochloric acid** from deep within the pits kills any microbes in swallowed food; other cells in the pits release **gastric lipase** which starts to breakdown lipids (fats) into fatty acids and **monoglycerides**. Proteins are broken down, into peptide chains, by **pepsin,** which when first released is in an inactive form (**pepsinogen**) to prevent it from digesting the stomach. Only when it is mixed with the stomach's acids does it become active. A lining of mucus protects the stomach's lining. Stomach acid also inactivates salivary amylase. Small amounts of water are absorbed by the stomach's lining.

The stomach has 3 muscle layers: longitudinal, circular and oblique. These 3 muscle layers churn and mix the food with gastric juices. After 3 to 4 hours the liquidized meal (called **chyme**) is released into the **duodenum** via the **pyloric sphincter** but only a small amount at a time.

The duodenum is the first of 3 sections of the small intestine. The next section is the **jejunum**, and the third is the **ileum**. The small intestine is made up of smooth muscle. Wave like *peristalsis*, created by the circular and longitudinal muscles of the smooth intestine push the chyme along the intestinal tract.

In the duodenum chyme is mixed with bile from gallbladder and digestive enzymes (that break down carbohydrates, proteins and lipids) from the pancreas. The bile duct from the gallbladder and the pancreatic duct from the pancreas enter the duodenum called the **ampulla of Vater.**

In the small intestine **peptidases** break peptides into amino acids. Carbohydrates are broken down into simple sugars. These, together with fatty acids are absorbed into the bloodstream via the **villi,** tiny (up to 1mm) finger like projections on the lining of the small intestine. These greatly increase the surface of the intestine by about 500 times, so absorption is more efficient. Some water is also absorbed together with the fat soluble vitamins A, D, E, water soluble vitamins B, C and the minerals iron, sodium, calcium.

At the end of the small intestine there is valve to control the flow of liquidized food in the first part of the large intestine, the ascending colon. This valve is called the

ileocecal valve. About 2 litre of liquid pass through this valve each day into the first part of the large intestine.

Water, sodium and chloride are absorbed from the chyme into bloodstream and lymph. The faeces become less watery. From glands in the colon potassium and bicarbonate are secreted into the faeces. There are billions of **symbiotic micro-organisms** (so-called friendly bacteria) that break down plant fibre that human enzymes cannot digest. They also produce vitamins K and B; and the gasses methane, hydrogen, carbon dioxide and hydrogen sulphide. When faeces are excreted at least 1/3 of their weight is composed of these bacteria.

The large intestine (ascending, transverse and descending colon) is not smooth but split into sections or pockets called **haustra** linked by longitudinal bands of muscle called taeni coli. The net effect of these muscles is to collate and compress the faeces. Faecal material moves more slowly through the large intestine than it does through the small intestine. This allows reabsorption of up to 2 litres (4 ¼ pints) of water every day. The final colonic section is the sigmoid colon, which makes an s-shaped band to the rectum, which leads finally to the anus. The rectum is about 5cm long and is normally empty, except just before and during defecation.

All nutrients gained from the digestion of food enter the hepatic portal vein. This is a network of veins from the stomach and intestines which merges and then enters the liver. It is nutrient rich and oxygen poor. In the liver branches of the hepatic vein enter liver lobules. These lobules process nutrients and produce bile which is transported and stored in the gallbladder. The hepatic vein then enters a central vein in the lobules which drains blood back to the inferior vena cava.

It can take food normally 24 hours to travel the entire length of the digestive tract, which is approximately 9 meters (30 feet) long from the mouth to the anus.

Chapter 12

Never skip on breakfast
It's your best friend!
(Plus a bit on the glycaemic index)

Breakfast not only kick starts your metabolism, but those who indulge in it are just as likely, if not more so, to lose weight than those who skip it. Ignoring these morning hunger pangs can also lead to more sluggish energy levels for the remainder of the day.

Different people have different dietary needs. Diabetics need to control their blood sugar levels. Some may need to control the amount of calories that they intake, either to lose weight or to gain weight. There is something called the **glycaemic index** (GI) which shows how fast food is broken down to increase the body's blood sugar. Low glycaemic index foods increase blood sugar slowly; high glycaemic index foods increase the blood sugar quickly.

Examples of low GI

Shredded Wheat has a low glycaemic Index (GI) which helps to control your appetite by releasing sugar into the blood stream at a more gradual pace.

Porridge Oats are high in magnesium, vitamin B1, and fibre, all of which are capable of lowering LDL (bad) cholesterol, while also having a low GI. Adding honey will not only add a sweet flavour to your porridge, but has also been shown to boost energy levels and raise serotonin, a mood-elevating hormone. Eating a small bowl of porridge, with sliced banana and a honey, an hour or so before a run for example will give you a slow, steady supply of fuel for a while.

Example of high GI

Sports drinks are designed to boost blood sugar (glucose) levels quickly. During prolonged exercise, like long distance running or cycling, glucose will be used up quickly and needs to be replaced whilst exercising.

Try to avoid breakfasts that are high in saturated fat. However, the occasional naughty breakfast is good for soul!

Sometime before a moderate run (about 5 to 8 miles), I used to have a Shredded Wheat and fruit smoothie. And after the run, Porridge Oats and All Bran. Indeed, sometimes I would have a protein and fruit smoothie. When doing longer runs I might have scrambled eggs on toast before the run, then a large protein and fruit smoothies afterwards. I found out very quickly that trying to run on an empty stomach is not a good idea.

Some people, when they wake up in the morning, say "It's too early for breakfast before I go to work!" Then they get there and find it hard to concentrate, they feel tired and so on. Also this can have the effect of telling your body to store lipids and breakdown muscle mass for energy! And for those who have a high glycaemic index breakfast, their sugar levels increase quite quickly then plummet a few hours later. And don't forget that your body has to produce insulin for your cells to take in your large intake of blood sugar produced by the high glycaemic index food. Then you might not eat for several hours but the high insulin produced is still letting cells consume the glucose at a high rate. This high oscillating blood sugar level could lead to diabetes. Plus, any excess calories that are not used up simply get turned into lipids and is squirrelled away in your fat cells; but then you still feel hungry a bit later with your fat cells saying "Yum, thanks for the extra lipids!" And the end result is that you put on more fat while still feeling hungry!

Or, you might choose a low GI breakfast which produces a fairly constant level of glucose, which is just enough for your energy needs, insulin levels stay about constant and your fat cells sit there sulking because they don't get any more lipids! (Poor little things!). And if you use more calories than you take in your weight will be reduced. But a word of caution … work those muscles to stop them from being broken down for energy, while the lipid still sits there in your fat cells. It's harder for the body to metabolise fat than it is to metabolise protein.

Wake up and enjoy having a low GI breakfast!

Chapter 13

Diabetes, insulin and glucose

There are 2 types of diabetes, which are just called type 1 and type 2.

To understand what effect these have on your body we need to look at how cells in your body take up glucose, which enables you to have energy to do things. Without your body's cells being able to use glucose your body's cells will die. And, as we are all made of cells, we too will die.

In your body the pancreas produces insulin – in things called **beta cells** – which travels in the blood to cells and locks on to them. The cells in response to insulin are then able to take up glucose and, once in the cell, is converted to energy. Normally the insulin is regulated automatically in response to intake of food.

What is glucose?

Glucose is simply blood sugar. The body makes glucose from proteins, fats, and in the largest part carbohydrates. Glucose is basically a plain sugar (monosaccharide), it is a key carbohydrate in biology. The living cell converts it into a form of energy which the cell can utilize. This energy is **adenosine triphosphate** (ATP).

Type 1 diabetes

This occurs because the beta cell on the pancreas are destroyed by the body's own immune system. The insulin receptor points on the cells are working normally and are waiting for insulin, but there is insufficient insulin in the blood for cells to absorb glucose. Type 1 diabetics need insulin with food for their cells to be able to absorb glucose.

Type 2 diabetes

This differs from type 1 in that there is insulin in the blood from the beta cells but the receptors do not recognize the insulin and so are not able to absorb the glucose. Regular exercise and a healthy diet can help to reduce symptoms. Condition is ongoing and may need medication to help insulin lock onto cells. Those with type 2 diabetes are prone to high levels of cholesterol, atherosclerosis and high blood pressure.

Symptoms of diabetes

These include weight loss, frequent passing of urine, being more thirsty than normal, tiredness, regular infection like thrush and itching around the genitals.

Normal blood sugar range

Normal blood sugar is in the range 4.4 mm/litre to 6.8 mm/litre but can rise slightly after a meal. As mentioned, every time we eat our blood sugar increases. And as time passes and all the food has been digested, we're still active and burning up glucose so our blood sugar starts to drop. When our blood sugar drops too low it's called **hypoglycaemia**; when your blood sugar goes to high it's called **hyperglycaemia**.

Hypoglycaemia and hyperglycaemia

Symptoms of a hypoglycaemic attack (very low blood sugar, less than 4mm/litre) are: shaking, trembling, sweating, excessive hunger, pallor, irritability, rapid heartbeat, palpitations, headaches, fuzzy thinking, dizziness, feeling light headed, confusion, drowsiness, aggression, slurred speech, blurred vision, feeling cold, prickly skin, seizures; in extreme cases loss of consciousness, even death.

For a quick response take a handful of dried fruit, glass of fruit juice, or glucose tablet.

Symptoms of a Hyperglycaemic attack (very high blood sugar, greater than 6.8mm/litre) include: vomiting, stomach pain, rapid breathing, and breath that smells of ketones – like pear drops or nail varnish. If untreated quickly can lead to coma or death.

Long term complications include damage to kidneys (**nephropathy**), eyes (**cataracts**, **glaucoma**, **retinopathy**), nerves (**neuropathy**), skin problems, loss of limbs.

Before exercising:

Always consult a doctor before starting any exercise if you have diabetes.

Type 1 diabetics are insulin injection dependent. So before exercise it's important to get the right amount of insulin in to the blood stream: too much could result in a hypoglycaemic attack; and too little could result in a hyperglycaemic attack.

Low impact, low intensity aerobic exercise is good for diabetics because working muscle cells will take up more glucose than inactive ones. Could help with weight loss in type2 diabetes. Exercise reduces stress leaves. Cardiovascular exercise will help the heart and lungs become stronger; using weights will strengthen muscles.

Chapter 14

The heart

(Cardiovascular system)

The heart is duel pump which moves blood around the body in a controlled rhythm. It has four chambers. Each pump has two chambers; and each has valves to control the flow of blood.

Below is my drawing of the heart..

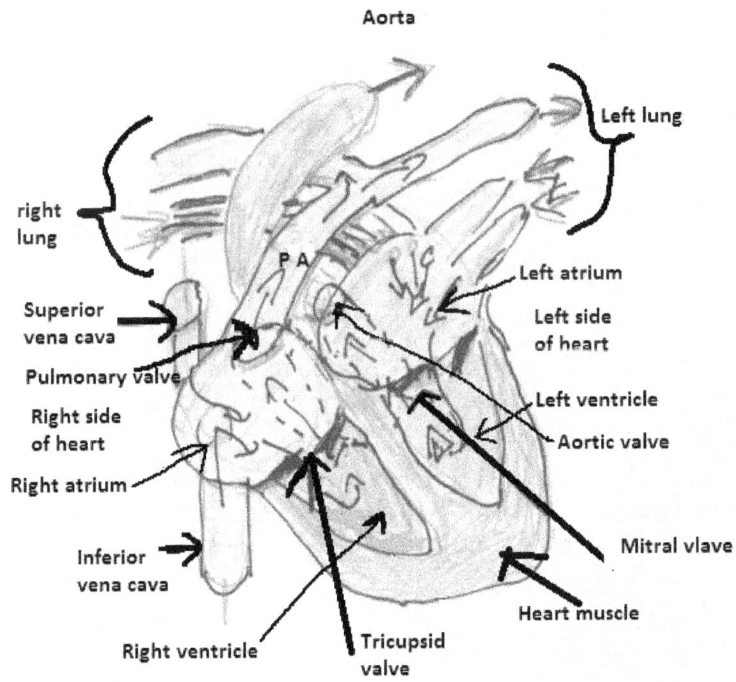

The aorta carries oxygenated blood to every part of the body – cells, tissues etc. On the right side of the heart we have the superior vena cava which brings de-oxygenated blood from the upper body to the right atrium; and the inferior vena cava which brings de-oxygenated blood from the lower half of the body back to the right atrium

Going to the left and right lungs we have the **pulmonary artery** (P A in the drawing) which take de-oxygenated blood to the lungs.

From the lungs oxygenated blood flows to the left atrium.

The heart's natural pacemaker is called the **sinoatrial node** which is located in the right atrium. There is another node in the right atrium, and this sends electrical signals through the heart to make it contract, that is to beat, and this is called the **atrioventricular node**.

The natural beating frequency of an adult's heart is 100 beats per minute; this is called its intrinsic rate. In the brain stem there is a region called the **cardio regulatory centre**. It is this control unit that sets the heart's resting heart rate to about 70 beats per minute. The resting heart is influenced by hormones such as **adrenaline** and during activity or stress. Caffeine also affects it. Athletes normally have a much lower resting heart rate. A resting heart rate less than 60 beats per minute is considered to be an athlete's resting heart rate.

Systole is the term given to describe the contraction of the heart, which pushes blood out of the heart. All 4 chambers undergo systole.

Diastole refers to the period when the chambers of the heart relax and fills with blood. **Ventricular diastole** is the period when the verticals are relaxing; similarly, **atrial diastole** is the period when the atria are relaxing and filling with blood.

There are four phases to one heartbeat. Below is a description of the four phases.

1. **Phase 1**. This is where de-oxygenated blood under low pressure flows from the inferior and superior vena cava to the right atrium; and at the same time the left atrium fills with oxygenated blood from the lungs. Some blood flows down into both ventricles at this time to about 80 percent capacity. This is the relaxation phase or the **late diastole.**

2. **Phase 2**. This is where both the left and right atrium contract to push blood down into the left and right ventricles, through the mitral and tricuspid valves. This called the **atrial systole**, which is triggered by a pulse from the sinoatrial node (By the way, the word atria is the plural of word atrium.)

3. **Phase 3**. Contraction of the ventricles or **ventricular systole**. This is the power stroke of the heartbeat. The muscle walls of the ventricles contract and force blood into the aortic valve and pulmonary valve. Once the contraction has stopped the valves snap shut.

4. **Phase 4**. The walls of the ventricles begin to relax. This is the early diastole. As the ventricles expand, because the ventricular muscles are relaxing, the high pressure in the arteries compared to low pressure in the ventricles causes the aortic and pulmonary valves remain closed. As ventricular pressure in the tricuspid and mitral valves decrease they once again open, allowing blood to enter from the main veins.

Blood pressure is the term given to describe force on the walls of blood vessels exerted by circulating blood flow. The term usually refers to arterial pressure – i.e. the pressure in the larger arteries (those which take blood away from the heart).

Arterial pressure is measured with a **sphygmo-manometer.**

Blood pressure is measured in **millimetres of mercury** (mmHg). Electronic blood pressure meters do not use mercury. However, the reading is still in mmHg.

Blood pressure reading has 2 values:

Systolic (peak pressure)

--- **over** ---

Diastolic (minimum pressure)

An example would be 120 / 75.

Average blood pressure reading is 120/70 to 135/ 80

High blood pressure (140/90) is another term for **hypotension**.

The term **cardiac output** refers to the amount of blood the heart can pump per minute. It is defined as

(Heart rate) x (stroke volume).

The term **maximum heart rate** refers to the absolute maximum beats per minute that your heart can achieve during maximal physical exertion.

One formula used to predict a person's maximum heart rate is

220 – (their age) beats per minute.

Oxygenated blood needs to be delivered to every cell in the body. Without sufficient blood pressure cells may not receive enough oxygen to work properly. But if the pressure is too high it could cause damage to some of the body's organs.

4 things that can raise blood pressure are:

- Smoking
- Being overweight
- Taking in large quantities of sodium

- Alcohol can cause blood pressure to rise in some people.

Resting heart rate is defined as the slowest beats per minute when your body is at rest. It is often used as an indication of how fit a person is: the more athletic a person is the lower the resting heart rate. An average person's resting heart rate is 60 -70 beats per minute; but athletes have a lower rate. **Bradycardia** is the term given to a person's resting heart rate which is below 60 beats per minute (bpm); and which is also referred to as an athlete's heart rate.

And lastly: deliver refers to the delivery of oxygen to the body's cells; extract refers to the removal of waste elements from the cells: carbon dioxide and water.

Chapter 15
Arteries, veins and capillaries

Under your skin there is a network of tubes which allows blood to flow around your body. These are called **arteries**, **veins** and **capillaries**. They range in diameter from large, like the aorta, down to the capillaries, very tiny in diameter which allow oxygen, nutrients etc. to pass into cells; and waste products to be removed from the cells.

Arteries are the largest and carry oxygen and glucose to every cell in the body. Veins normally carry oxygen depleted blood back to the heart.

There are two definitions relating to the movement and exchange of oxygen, nutrients and waste. They are: *deliver* refers to the delivery of oxygen and nutrients to the body's cells; *extract* refers to the removal of waste elements from the cells: carbon dioxide and water.

There are 2 main components of blood, and they are **red blood cells** and **plasma** (55% of total volume).

> **Red blood cells**: also known as **erythrocytes**; their primary function is to carry oxygen to all cells from the lungs and to carry carbon dioxide to the lungs.

> **White blood cells**, on the other hand, are known as **leukocytes**. They protect the body from bacteria. These blood cells are infarct colourless. There are many different forms of white blood cells; and each fight bacteria etc. in different ways.

Platelets are also known as **thrombocytes**. They are fragments of cells, which don't contain a nucleus, that fuse together to stop leaks in the cardiovascular system.

Many larger veins, like those in the legs, have a valve which prevents the back flow of blood, which is under relatively low pressure, from being pulled back down by gravity. Veins are more flexible than arteries and are much thinner. Blood in veins flows slowly and smoothly.

Chapter 16
Heart disease

To begin with, there are many different types of heart disease: **stroke, angina, congestive heart failure, heart attack (myocardial infarction), atherosclerosis (arteriosclerotic vascular disease)**. What follows is a brief look at each one.

Stroke.

Blood vessels in the brain may become blocked or may haemorrhage so that blood, which contains oxygen and nutrients, fails to reach the brain cells. Damage to the brain quickly follows and results in loss of function to the part of the body that is controlled by the damaged area of the brain.

When a stroke is caused by blocked artery or arteries this is called an **ischaemic stroke.**

When a stroke is caused by bleeding in or around the brain it is called **a haemorrhagic stroke.**

There are two types of haemorrhagic stroke:

1. Intra-cerebral haemorrhage in which there is bleeding inside the brain itself.

2. Subarachnoid haemorrhage in which a blood vessel bursts and bleeds into the subarachnoid space, which surrounds the brain.

Angina.

This is the result of the heart muscle not receiving enough blood due to **atherosclerosis**, (narrowing of the arteries), during intensive exercise. Symptoms are an intense pain behind the breast bone and down the arms, more often the left. Sometimes a constriction in the throat and jaw can be felt. These symptoms usually subside within 15 minutes once at rest. Medication can be taken to relax and widen the arteries to reduce the effects of angina.

Congestive Heart Failure.

This refers to heart's inability to pump blood around the body smoothly and in a controlled manor. It commonly refers to both left and right side of the heart. Failure can be described as acute (coming on suddenly) or chronic (developing over time).

Acute heart failure is due to trauma of the heart due to heart attack or valve failure. It results in wheezing and breathlessness, sweaty pale skin and coughing that brings up sputum. Chronic heart failure is a long term problem with many causes: coronary heart disease, continuous high blood pressure, valve or rhythm disorder, obstructive pulmonary disease. In the left side chronic heart failure, blood is not pumped out of the heart as fast as it enters so blood begins to back up to the lungs, causing congestion. Fluid begins to build up in the lungs; oxygen is not absorbed efficiently resulting in breathlessness, coughing and fatigue. In right sided chronic heart failure blood is not pumped to the lungs as fast as it enters the heart, so again blood backs up in the main veins. Increased venous pressure forces fluid out of the capillaries and into tissues. This could cause swelling (oedema) in the ankles and lower back. May also include nausea and fatigue.

Heart Attack (myocardial infarction)

When the supply of blood is interrupted to some part of the heart causing heart cells to die, a myocardial infraction occurs. This is due to the heart disease atherosclerosis where the inner walls of the arteries narrow, restricting blood flow (this is called **ischaemia**). A blood clot (**thrombus**) can form cutting of supply of blood, causing a heart attack.

Atherosclerosis (Arteriosclerotic Vascular Disease)

This is a condition in which the arterial walls thicken due to fatty deposits and cholesterol. These substances get into the lining of the arteries at sites which have microscopic damage, and there accumulate to form athermanous plaque, on top of which is a fibrous cap. The plaques narrow the space (lumen) within the arteries causing disturbances in the blood flow, which may cause eddies and these could lead to clots forming. There are two types of atherosclerosis: arteriosclerosis, this is the hardening of any medium or large arteries; arteriolosclerosis, this is the hardening of arterioles (small arteries).

Numerous things in everyday life can increase the risk of developing heart disease. These include: smoking, heavy drinking, eating foods high in saturated fat, not taking adequate exercise, stress, obesity, high blood cholesterol. A point worth noting is people with diabetes, especially type II diabetes, and heart problems are more likely to have a fatal heart attack.

Exercise for those who have a heart condition

Those who are suffering from arteriosclerosis must get clearance from their GP to start an exercise program because of the risk of the hardened arteriole walls failing.

Whatever the medical condition you may have, you need to provide documented proof that you are fit enough to begin even moderate exercise.

There are two main benefits of exercise to be gained by those with heart disease: reduced blood pressure; reduced cholesterol.

Short term affects that exercise can have on the cardiovascular system are:

- Reducing LDL cholesterol and fat levels.

- Improved blood circulation and therefore improved circulation of nutrients, gasses and hormones.

- Promoting muscle growth by tearing muscles so that they might be rebuilt stronger. Muscle growth requires extra protein, so one's diet has to be modified to take to take this into account.

- Getting that feel good factor.

    o Exercise lowers stress hormones like cortisol; and release the body's feel good chemicals – endorphins.

    o In a gym environment you may start to feel more relaxed and confident and integrate with other people around you and become less self-conscious.

Long term affect that exercise can have on the heart:

- Like all muscles the heart gets stronger as a result of exercise.

- Reducing the chances of a myocardial infraction (heart attack).

- Regular exercise keeps the arteries flexible.

- Keeping blood pressure within normal limits.

- Reducing the risk of developing type II diabetes.

- Maintaining bone density and strong skeletal muscles.

Chapter 17
The liver and what
It does for you

The function of the liver is to:

- Process nutrients gained from food, the storage of these nutrients.

- Circulation of vitamins and, minerals.

- The construction of complex molecules such as enzymes.

- Bile production (which breaks down fats).

- Synthesizes amino acids.

- Maintains blood glucose level (by converting fat and proteins into glucose).

- Detoxification of the blood.

- Protein synthesis (blood clotting proteins and plasma).

- Mineral storage (such as iron and copper) and vitamin storage (fat soluble vitamins A, D, E, K together with B12).

- Recycling of old red blood cells.

- Blood waste disposal.

- There are hundreds of liver cells that make up the liver. These cells are called lobules. Each functions on its own and contributes to the overall functioning of the liver. So if a lobule becomes damaged the liver is still able to function, although not at 100%.

- Alcohol abuse biggest destroyer of liver lobules. The live can repair itself to an extent. But persistent alcohol abuse will permanently damage the cells of the liver lobules, resulting in cirrhosis and this can be life threatening.

Chapter 18
Thyroid gland and
Parathyroid glands

The thyroid is an endocrine gland (these glands secrete hormones directly into the blood rather than through a duct). It controls how quickly the body uses energy, metabolism, by secreting 2 hormones called thyroxine and triiodothyronine. Iodine and the amino acid tyrosine are required to make thyroid hormone; both of which are present in the diet. Thyroid hormone controls how sensitive the body should be other hormones and controls body weight and heart rate. Unlike other endocrine glands it can store its hormones. The thyroid gland is controlled by the hypothalamus and pituitary gland.

The parathyroid glands, usually 4, are small glands found at the back of the thyroid. They release parathormone (PTH), which raises the level of calcium in the blood. PTH acts on the kidneys to prevent calcium loss, acts on the bones to absorb or release calcium and acts on the intestines to absorb calcium. Another hormone, calcitonin, lowers the level of calcium in the blood. And, don't forget, for calcium to be absorbed vitamin D needs to be present in the diet.

An under active thyroid (**hypothyroidism**) causes the slowing down of the body's functions. Iodine deficiency could be the cause of the condition. New mothers may also develop the condition, of which 1 in 5 may develop permanent symptoms.

Symptoms include:

- Dry and/or pale skin.

- Feeling tired and sleeping a lot.

- Feeling the cold easily.

- Coarse, thinning hair and brittle nails.

- Paleness.

- Depression.

- Goitre.

- Weight gain and water retention.

- Mental slowing.

An over active thyroid (**hyperthyroidism**) relates to the speeding up of the metabolism. Possible causes include: the entire gland overproducing hormones (termed Graves Disease), thyroiditis (inflammation of the thyroid) low iodine levels.

Symptoms include:

- Sleeping poorly.

- Losing weight although having a good appetite.

- Feeling tired.

- Having more frequent bowel movements or diarrhoea.

- Shortness of breath.

- Swelling of the thyroid gland.

- Feeling nervous, emotional or irritable.

- Increased heart rate or palpitations.

Chapter 19

Your kidneys and what
They do for you

They are essential in many regulatory roles, especially the urinary system and also serve in **homeostatic functions** (property of a system that regulates its internal environment and tends to maintain a stable, constant condition of properties such as temperature or pH).

They remove nitrogenous waste from the blood and excrete urine. They are located in the small of the back.

Every 45 minutes they filter out about 4.5 litres of the water content of the blood. Glucose, minerals and needed water is returned to the body by reabsorption. The reaming fluid and waste pass into collecting ducts, flowing to the ureter and bladder as urine. Each kidney has over one million functioning units (*nephrons*) involved in the process of filtration and reabsorption. The kidneys also secrete *renin*, an enzyme involved in blood pressure regulation.

Renal failure or kidney failure.

This refers to partial or complete loss of kidney function. This causes reduced urine output and blood chemical imbalance. Damage to various kidney structures can occur from chemical exposure, major loss of blood, hypotension, severe burns, crush injury, severe kidney infections, diabetes, renal artery or urinary tract blockage and liver disease.

Kidney failure can lead to complications such as **pulmonary oedema** (relating to build up of excessive fluid in the tissues in the heart), high potassium levels and heart failure. If the blood becomes too acidic bones can lose calcium and nerves can degenerate.

The kidneys can sustain life until they lose about 90% of their functional ability. If one is removed the other increases in size and function to compensate.

Failure of both kidneys usually requires dialysis or kidney transplant.

Kidney stones what are they?

They are a mass of minerals and organic matter that may form in the kidney.

Urine contains many salts in solution, and a low fluid volume or high mineral concentration can cause theses salts to precipitate and grow and ultimately to form stones.

Large stones can block the flow of urine, be the focus of infection, or cause **renal colic** (painful spasms). They can obstruct the urinary system at various parts.

Treatment may involve drugs to dissolve the stones or ultrasound (**lithotripsy**), or removal of large ones by surgery.

To avoid getting kidney stones, make sure you drink plenty of water each day to avoid becoming dehydrated. It is very important to keep your urine diluted to avoid waste products forming into kidney stones. Refer to the section water requirements for more information.

As a brief note, you can tell how diluted your urine is by looking at its colour. The darker your urine is, the more concentrated it is. Your urine is usually a dark yellow colour in the morning because it contains a build-up of waste products that your body has produced overnight. But normally it should be a lot lighter.

Chapter 20
Respiratory system or breathing

There is more to breathing then just using your lungs. A lot of different muscles are used in breathing. But the main muscle used is the diaphragm. It separates the thoracic cavity (the area enclosed by the ribs) from the abdominal cavity. The diaphragm is a sinewy, dome-shaped, wide structure. It is critical for normal breathing. During inhalation the diaphragm contracts and in doing so increases the thoracic cavity. Intra-thoracic pressure is reduced and this draws air into the lungs. The oesophagus goes through the diaphragm as does the major blood vessels.

Between the ribs there are pairs of muscles called the **intercostals**. The external intercostals muscles (we may call them inspiratory intercostals) also play a role in the enlargement of the thoracic cavity, and so help you to take in air. When the diaphragm relaxes air in the lungs is exhaled by elastic recoil of the lungs and the tissues lining the thoracic cavity. The abdominal muscle acts an **antagonist** paired with the diaphragm's contraction and so aids exhalation. The internal intercostals (or expiratory intercostals) also work to squeeze air out of the lungs.

So we know that the main muscles used in breathing are the diaphragm and the intercostal muscles. But there are other muscles in other parts of the body that are important as well. These are called the *accessory* muscles. And these are listed below.

- The **scalene** *muscles* – 3 pairs of muscles in the lateral neck

1. Scalenus Anterior
2. Scalenus Medius
3. Scalenus Posterior

- The **sternocleidomastoid** muscle, is a muscle in the superficial layers of the anterior part of the neck. It acts to rotate and flex the head.

- The wings of the nose, which cause nasal flaring.

- The small muscles in the neck and head also help with breathing.

OK, so you know which muscles are used in breathing but what happens to the air you breathe in? Well when you breathe in, air travels down the bronchial tubes to the lungs where it enters microscopic sacs called **alveoli**. Once there the oxygen in the air is able to diffuse into blood capillaries and from there enter the circulatory system. This system allows oxygen to travel around your body to cells in something called **haemoglobin**, which is a protein that is red in colour, and which contains iron. Once the cells receive oxygen they can then do **cellular respiration**... a term used to describe work done by different parts of the cell.

By-products of cellular respiration are carbon-dioxide and water. They are transported back to the alveoli to be expelled as the air you breathe out.

Another term is the **respiratory rate** and this is the rate at which you breathe in and out per minute. A normal healthy adult's resting respiratory rate is about 12 per minute.

Chapter 21
Asthma

A large proportion of people get asthma; but what is it?

It's a respiratory condition marked by spasms in the bronchi of the lungs, causing difficulty in breathing, by constricting the airways. Wheezing, coughing, tightening of the chest, breathlessness are symptoms of asthma, which can range from mild to life-threatening. It usually results from an allergic reaction or other forms of hypersensitivity. Dust, pollen, animal fur, or other particles in the air can trigger an asthmatic attack.

Inhalers which are used by asthmatics help to open the airways.

Different types of light aerobic exercises may help to reduce the symptoms of asthma. Exercising will strengthen the heart and lungs and will increase oxygen intake. Examples:

- o Static cycling.
- o Walking on the treadmill.
- o Moderate use of resistance training once or twice a week.

However, always consult a specialist before starting to exercise if you have any underling health issues.

Chapter 22

In which we have a brief note on the different types of organic cells

And a very simple over view of energy production

In your cells (cellular respiration)

There are more than 200 different types of cell in the human body. Ranging from skin cells to nerve cells, optic nerves, muscle cells, brain cells, fat cells and connective tissue etc. Well you get the picture. But they all have one thing in common: they all need energy and oxygen to function; and without which they die. One cell doesn't change into another. Fat cells don't become muscles cells for example.

Human cells are called **eukaryotic cells**; so are the cells of plants, animals and fungi. These have a nucleus that contains DNA, contain **organelles** – we'll talk about those later – in a jelly like substance called the **cytoplasm**.

Another type of cell is the **prokaryotic cell**. These don't have a nucleus that contain DNA. Their DNA is in the cytoplasm of the cell, and they don't have any organelles.

Eukaryotic and prokaryotic cells have a few things in common:

- They have cell walls made of proteins and lipids. This is called the **plasma membrane** or **cytoplasmic membrane.**

- They have **cytoplasm,** a jelly like substance enclosed by the cell membrane.

- All cells contain DNA.

- All cells make proteins.

As mentioned earlier, eukaryotic cells contain things called organelles. There are different types of organelles that perform different functions within the cells. But all work together as a unit so the cells can perform work. This is called the **endomembrane system**. Each organelle is enclosed in a membrane.

Here is a list of the organelles in a typical eukaryotic cell:

- **Nucleus** containing the cell's DNA.

- **Golgi apparatus**. This puts proteins into packets to be transported out of the cell.

- **Centriole**. Used in cell division.

- **Mitochondria**. This is the cell's power station. It produces something called **adenosine triphosphate** (ATP), which powers all the cell's activity. We'll talk about ATP later.

- **Lysosome**. This is where old cell parts are broken down and where macromolecules (such as proteins, polysaccharides and nucleic acids), and microorganisms are broken down (digested).

- **Microfilaments** (actin and myosin) used to contract muscle cells. These are proteins.

- **Cytoskeletal proteins** that give the cell shape.

- **Endoplasmic reticulum**. Two types: rough endoplasmic reticulum (RER) and smooth endoplasmic reticulum (SER). Proteins are made in the RER, and lipids are made in the SER.

- **Ribosomes**. These are attached to the RER.

- **Vesicles**. These carry molecules around the cell, bring products into the cell and products to the cell wall.

- **Peroxisomes**. They help to breakdown lipids. And those in the liver breakdown poisons like ethanol form alcohol.

Blood is made of white cells **(leukocytes)**, red blood cells **(erythrocytes)** and **platelets (thrombocytes)**. Red blood cells don't have mitochondria, are rich in haemoglobin, don't have a nucleus. About 2.4 million erythrocytes are produced in the body every second. They develop in the bone marrow and circulate the body for about 100 to 120 days then they are recycled by **macrophages** – a type of white blood cell. About 200 billion erythrocytes are destroyed every day by the spleen and must be replaced. White blood cells are involved in the defence of the body – the body's immune system. Unlike red blood cells they have a nucleus. Platelets are cells that circulate the body and react to bleeding. They clump together to stop the flow of blood. They do not have a nucleus.

Cellular respiration is energy production in the eukaryotic cells which takes place in the mitochondria with oxygen. The job of the mitochondria is to produce **adenosine triphosphate** (ATP). Every function that takes place in the body needs ATP to work: producing enzymes, contracting muscles, looking at the world around us, utilizing food, thinking. ATP is not energy in itself but acts like a battery that holds potential energy, which is then moved from one place to another. The mitochondria produce ATP by combining a phosphate to **adenosine diphosphate** (ADP). ATP has three phosphate groups while ADP has two. It is the extra phosphate that is used to make things happen within the cell. When ATP releases a phosphate energy is released and work can be done. The production of ATP itself requires ATP. When oxygen is available one molecule of glucose produces about thirty 36 ATP Molecules. Lipids can also be broken down to produce ATP, as can muscle. There are several stages within the mitochondria in order for it to produce ATP. The first step is to break down glucose; and this is done in the cytoplasm of the cell. This is called **glycolysis**. The result of glycolysis is two molecules of **pyruvat*e*** and two ATP. The pyruvate enters the mitochondria. The next stage is the formation of **acetyl coenzyme A.** Next is the **Krebs cycle**, which turns acetyl coenzyme A into **oxaloacetic acid** which then turns into **citric acid**, which produces 2 ATP and hydrogen, which is later used in the end cycle. And finally, in the end cycle the hydrogen is split into a proton and electron. The electron powers ATP syntheses, and the proton is oxidised to from water; and about 32 ATP are produced. This is called the aerobic energy system, as it uses oxygen. The by-product of this carbon-dioxide and water.

When exercising, muscle cells require huge amounts of ATP to make them contract. The advantage of using the aerobic energy system is it doesn't produce lactic acid, produces a large amount of ATP. However, when breaking down fatty acids, it needs about 15% more oxygen than breaking down glucose.

Creatine is the product of protein metabolism which is made naturally in our bodies to supply energy. It is mainly produced in the liver from the amino acids arginine, glycine and methionine. It is transported in the blood to muscle cells where it is combined with phosphate to produce **phosphocreatine** (PC) and stored in the **sarcoplasm** of the muscle. Once there it can be broken down to provide energy to synthesise ATP. This provides large amounts of energy. PC can be replenished quickly, about 50% in 30 seconds and about 100% in 3 minutes. This is called the **ATP -PC system.** Some disadvantages are: it doesn't last very long, only happens when oxygen is present, only produces 1 ATP and you need to be working as hard as you can – maximum effort.

The brain, heart and muscles cells require vast amounts of energy to function. This is proved by phosphocreatine.

The last energy producing system is called **anaerobic glycolysis**. This is where glycogen (glucose in form that is stored in the liver and muscles) is broken down into molecules of glucose, then further broken down into pyruvic acid; and this produces 2 ATP. Because there is no oxygen present, lactic acid is produced which causes cramp in the muscles, and this occurs in the sarcoplasm of the muscle. The advantage of this system is that ATP can be produced quickly, providing extra bursts of energy – say a sprint when running or cycling as hard as you can. But this system only produces a small amount of energy and only lasts for a maximum of about 1 minute.

Chapter 23

Common illnesses
And ailments

Not many people are at an ideal weight for their size. Some are a little underweight, some are a lot underweight; some are overweight, and some are very overweight.

It is harder for someone who is overweight to lose weight than it is for someone who is underweight wishing to gain weight.

Being seriously underweight poses its own problems to the individual. Worst case can lead to damage to the body's internal organs.

But being overweight has many disadvantages:

- Potential high blood pressure.

- Developing type 2 diabetes.

- Heart problems.

- May lead to an increase in sleep apnoea.

- Weak pelvic/abdominal muscles leading to poor posture and back pain.

- Excess fat in the body makes walking, sitting and breathing harder.

- Self-confidence may also be an issue for some.

3 other medical conditions connected with being overweight:

- Higher level of LDL (bad cholesterol).

- May lead to gallstones.

- Osteoarthritis, due to increased pressure on joints.

For those who are overweight but wishing to lose weight a safe weekly weight loss would be 1 to 2 pounds a week. A combination of cardiovascular, like fast walking or cross training, together with resistance training, weights, is best for burning those stubborn pounds off. But exercising is only half of the story. The other half being diet.

Frequency and duration of exercise would depend on your level of fitness. As your confidence and stamina improves, the frequency and duration of exercise could be increased. However, don't overdo it. Listen to your body.

Arthritis.

There are two types of arthritis are: **osteoarthritis** and **rheumatoid arthritis.**

- In osteoarthritis it's the normal wear and tear of a joint, due to age, injury, infection or obesity that causes the articular cartilage to degenerate, the synovial membrane to become inflamed and the gap between the bones to be reduced. In time the bone ends thicken and rub against each other. This may be just localised to one joint.

- In rheumatoid arthritis the body's own immune system makes antibodies that attack the body's own tissues, which includes the synovial membrane in joints. These antibodies can be detected in the blood. The antibody rheumatoid factor (RhF) is associated with rheumatoid arthritis. The condition affects the left and right side of the body at the same time.

Gentle exercises may help to keep the joints moving for someone with osteoarthritis. However, only start exercising with the go-ahead from a doctor. Here are a few exercises:

- **Range of motion** (ROM). Joints maintain their range of motion by being moved, so it vital to keep joints moving with dynamic stretching.

- **Strength training exercises.** All these keep the muscles around the joint strong.

  o Isometric – where the joint angle and muscle length do not change during muscle fibre contraction

  o Isotonic – where the muscle length and joint angle change during contraction.

- **Low impact cardiovascular** like cycling, swimming if possible.

  Avoid high impact cardiovascular like road running and heavy weights.

  In all the above heat maybe applied to the joint(s) prior to exercising.

However, for rheumatoid arthritis if joints flare up you should stop immediately.

Other common illnesses include asthma and diabetes. Refer to separate sections for information on these.

Chapter 24
Connective tissue

There are different types of connective tissue which perform specific tasks within the body: **ligaments** support joints, **tendons** to connect muscle to bone, **elastic cartilage** (which is light weight, flexible and strong), of which is the type that holds the larynx open. But all connective tissue types are developed from the same jelly-like **ground substance,** or **extracellular matrix**, which is made up from salts, water, protein and carbohydrate. Within this jelly are various types of fibres and cells: collagen fibres for strength, **reticulin fibres** (reticular fibres) provide support, elastic fibres provide elasticity. White cells and macrophages fight infection, plasma cells to provide antibodies, and fat cells which are used as an energy store.

The three different types of connective tissue are:

- **Loose** – found in skin, surrounding blood vessels, nerves and organs.

- **Dense** --- bundles of parallel collagen fibres and fibroblasts (type of cell that manufactures collagen and extracellular matrix and plays a part in wound healing) found in tendons and ligaments.

    o   Tendons: connect muscle to bone via fibrous connective tissue. Their collagen fibres are arranged in parallel pattern which enables a high resistance in one direction as the muscles contracts.

    o   Ligaments: are fibrous connective tissue that connect bone to bone. These contain more elastin than tendons, and therefore more elastic. They provide stability for joints.

- **Cartilage** -- made from collagen and elastin fibres embedded in a matrix of glycoprotein and cells called chondrocytes which is found in small spaces. Cartilage covers the bone ends in many joints.
    - o **Cartilage has three subtypes**:
        - **Hyaline** – found at the end of long bones, structures in the ear and the nose.
        - **Elastic** – to maintain shape.
        - **Fibrous** – this the strongest type, it has dense collagen. It is found in the pelvis, skull, and vertebral discs.

- **Blood is classed as liquid connective tissue**.

- **Periostium** is connective tissue that surrounds bone.

- **Pericardium** is connective tissue that surrounds the heart.

- **Superficial fascia** is mainly loose connective tissue and fat cells that is found in most areas of the body, filling spaces between organs and glands, and binds the skin to muscles. It acts as a storage medium for fat and water. It is also a passage way for lymph, nerve and blood vessels.

- **Bursa**: a fluid filled sac that protects tendons and joints.

- **Perimysium** is connective tissue around a bundle (fascicle) of muscles cells.

- **Endomysium** is connective tissue between muscle fibres (individual muscles cells).

- **Epimysium** connective tissue that encapsulates a muscle.

Chapter 25

Bones, joints, the skeletal system
And osteoporosis

The skeletal system refers to the whole of the body working as a unit. The skeleton provides shape and protection for the body's soft tissue and organs and allows you to move. In the morrow of the bone, blood cells are manufactured to replace the ones that die each day in the body. Cells circulate the body for about 100 to 120 days before being destroyed by the liver. Millions of cells are produced every second. Bones are also a reservoir for calcium and minerals. White blood cells are also produced which destroys infection.

Bone is formed by ossification of **collagen fibres.**

Every day bone is broken down by **osteoclasts** and rebuilt by **osteoblasts**. Calcium is removed from the bone ever day to be used by muscles, as your muscles will not contract without calcium. It is vital that you take in calcium in your diet every day. Approximately 1000mg is recommended together with vitamins, particularly vitamin D.

In your body there are 4 bone groups, and they are:

- **Long bones**

    These work as levers and are found in the upper and lower part s of the body. They are longer than they are wide. They include the **femur, tibia, fibula, humerus, radius, ulna, metacarpals, metatarsals and phalanges.**

- **Short bones**

  They are found in the skeleton where strength, compactness is coupled with limited movement. They are defined as being approximately as wide as they are tall. They include the **carpals** in the wrist and *tarsals* in the ankle.

- **Flat bones**

  There are 2 main functions of these bones: protection over a large area; and broad surface area for muscle attachment. The **cranium, ilium, ribcage, sternum, scapular** and the **sacrum** are examples of flat bones.

- **Irregular bones**

  These have numerous functions in the body, one of which is multiple anchor points for skeletal muscles, another is the protection of nervous tissue and soft tissue support and attachment. Irregular bones which provide protection include the **vertebrae, sacrum, coccyx, temporal, sphenoid, ethmoid, zygomatic, maxilla, mandible, palatine, inferior nasal concha.** The trachea and pharynx gains support from irregular bones. Attachment bones include the **hyoid** bone, to which the tongue is connected.

There is a fifth type of bone called the **sesamoid bone** this bone is embedded in a tendon. An example of such is the kneecap (**patella**).

Joints

Fixed joints are those which do not move and are held together by ridged fibrous connective tissue. Example of such fixed joints are the joints between cranial bones.

Cartilaginous joints are of two types: in the first the joint is held together with **hyaline** cartilage, which is quite elastic, translucent and pearly in colour. They are found between the ribs and the sternum for example. The second type may have an internal cavity or nucleus as in the joints between the vertebrae of the spine.

Synovial joints are those which allow our limbs to move freely and give versatility. 4 classes of tissue make up the synovial joint. They are:

- o Cartilage.
- o Synovium.
- o Synovial fluid.
- o Ligaments and tendons.

These joints can work well for many decades if used often, but not over used. The ends of these bones are covered by a type of cartilage called an **articular cartilage,** which is compressible by a small amount and is smooth. Around the joint there is a covering called the **joint capsule**, made of strong connective tissue which is attached to the bone ends. Inside the capsule there is the synovial membrane which continuously secrets an oil like substance called **synovial fluid.** There are approximately 230 synovial joints in the body. Sometimes inflammation of the synovial membrane occurs and this is called **Synovitis.**

There are 6 different types of synovial joints:

1 plvot juint

There are 2 areas in the body that have pivot joints and they are the radius -- ulna and the occipital – axis joint. They have one bone encircled by another between which is a ligament disc.

2 Hinge joint

Allows movement mainly in one plane. At the joint one bone has convex surface and the other bone has a concave surface. An example would be the radius-ulna joint; and the finger joints. The knee is the largest hinge join in the human body.

3 Gliding Joint

In this type of joint the bones slide over each other, their surfaces being almost flat. Movement is limited by strong ligaments. An example would be between the tarsal bones of the ankle and between the carpal bones in the wrist.

4 Ball and Socket joint

Examples of the ball and socket joint are the humerus – scapula (arm to shoulder) joint and the pelvis – femur joint (hip to leg). In this type of joint one of the bones ends in a spheroidal shape and the other has a cup like cavity. The ball and socket joint gives the widest range of movement of all the synovial joints.

5 Saddle Joint

The main saddle joint is in the base of the thumb, the first metacarpal of the thumb; and the trapezium (wrist bone); and ankle joints. This type of joint enables you to grasp objects. Each bone at the joint has a convex – concave shape, like a horse saddle, that allows the bones to slide from side to side and back and forth but with limited rotation.

6 Ellipsoidal joints

An example of this type of joint is found at the radius – scaphoid (wrist) joint. These joints allow bending, extending, and rocking from side to side; but rotation is limited. One of these bones has an ovoid (egg shape) periphery which nestles in an ellipsoidal cavity.

There is a specialised joint called the *condylar* joint. This joint is like the hinge joint, but with a slight rotation allowing the joint to lock in an extended position. The knee joint is a condylar joint.

Flexion of a joint is a term given to the reduction of a joint angle. For example the elbow is flexed when the hand is brought to the shoulder. The neck can be flexed to bring the head to the chest; the knee can be flexed to bring the back of the foot to the buttocks.

Extension of a joint is a term given to the enlargement of an angle. For example the elbow joint is extended when the hand is taken away from the shoulder. The neck is extended when the head is taken away from the chest; the knee is flexed when the foot is taken away from the buttocks.

Hyperextension refers to the straightening of a joint beyond the normal limit of the joint extension. An example of this is the back hyperextension, which works the *erector spinae* muscles.

Circumduction refers to the circular movement of a limb.

Abduction refers to the movement of a limb away from the centre line of the body.

Adduction refers to the movement of a limb towards the centre line of the body.

Rotation refers to the limited movement of a limb about an axis in one direction; but cannot turn full circle. An example would be the forearm which rotates at the elbow to turn the palm of the hand from facing down

Osteoporosis

Osteoporosis is a condition that affects the bones, causing them to become weak and fragile and more likely to break (fracture). The word osteoporosis means porous bones. Under normal bone formation calcium, salts, phosphorus and other minerals are deposited on a framework of collagen fibres. This process is continuous as bone is also continuously broken down to provide calcium that the body to uses (muscles need calcium to contract); the process is also required for bone growth. Cells called *osteocytes* form collagen fibres and aid calcium deposition.

Calcium moves in canals between blood and bone in response to hormones. In osteoporotic bone the collagen-calcium framework is broken down much faster than it is built up, so the bone density decreases and so the bone becomes weak and prone to fractures.

All bones are formed from cartilage. The exception being the clavicle (collar bone) and some of the skull which *ossify* (turn to bone) directly from membrane. Long bones are made up of an outer covering called **periosteum**, the outer layer of which is the point of contact for muscles and contains fibroblasts, the inner (*cambium*) layer, containing **progenitor cells** which develop into **osteocytes**, provides good blood supply to the inner bone. Beneath the periosteum is a layer of compact bone (hard bone) -- the **cortical** bone -- which provides strength. Compact bone is composed of **osteons**, which are tightly packed concentric layers – or lamellae – that are formed by osteocytes. In the centre of these we have the **Haversian** canal that contain blood and lymph vessels. Beneath this we have the **spongy bone**, which is porous and light weight. In the centre of this spongy bone we have a canal called the **medullary cavity.** This spongy bone contains red bone marrow.

In an osteoporotic bone there is more spongy and less hard bone than normal. These fracture more easily than normal bone, mostly in the spine, wrist and hips but can affect other bones such as the arm or pelvis.

Exercises that could help maintain bone density include resistance training for all muscle groups, which encourage bone growth; and light cardiovascular, like cycling, swimming, walking. Exercise that could cause fracture include contact sports.

From about the age of 35, you gradually lose bone density. This is a normal part of ageing. But for some people it can lead to osteoporosis and an increased risk of fractures. Resistance training helps to reduce the chance of developing the condition. Other things that increase the risk of developing osteoporosis include: diseases of the hormone producing glands – such as an over active thyroid gland (hyperthyroidism), a family history of osteoporosis, long-term use of certain medications which affect bone strength or hormone levels, for example malabsorption problems, heavy drinking and smoking.

Deryck Britton

Chapter 26

The spine

In this section I cover different aspects of the spine, its muscles and what happens if the spine becomes damaged.

The spine consists of a total of 33 vertebrae. 24 are moveable leaving 9 that are none moveable (fused). The 24 moveable ones are divided into 3 sets. The first set is from the base of the skull to the collar bone; these are called the **cervical vertebrae** -- C1 to C7. C1 is called the *atlas* and C2 is called the *axis*. The next 12 are called the **thoracic vertebrae** T1 to T12, onto which are attached the ribs. The last 5 moveable vertebrae are called the **lumbar vertebrae** L1 to L5 – lower back vertebrae. Of the 9 fused vertebrae 5 are collectively known as the *sacrum* and 4 the *coccyx* (the last set of fused bone).

The seven cervical vertebrae, the ones from the base of the skull to the shoulder, are able to **flex** (i.e. tilt the head forward) by the use of the **sternocleidomastoid** muscle; **extend** (tilt backwards) the neck by the use of the **splenius capitis**. **Lateral flexion** (tilting the head to the shoulder) involves the use of the sternocleidomastoid and splenius muscles. The muscles used in lateral flexion are also used in rotation (turning the head from side to side).

The 12 thoracic and 5 lumbar move as one to **flex** the spine (bring the thorax closer to the pelvis) using the **rectus abdominis** and oblique muscles; extension / hyperextension by the use of **erector spinae** and trapezius (lower) muscles; **lateral flexion** (abduction), which is movement away from the midline of the body, is achieved by the **obliques**; **reduction** (adduction), straightening the spine from flexion and *rotation* uses the same muscles as for lateral flexion.

Separate vertebrae have between them a disc of fibrocartilage with a jelly-like core. These discs are called intervertebral discs. These allow the spinal column to flex and to act as a shock absorber. Each vertebra has a facet joint which determines the range of movement between vertebrae. Between each vertebrae are spring like ligaments that hold adjoining vertebrae in place. These limit movement and store energy for recoil.

The 5 fused vertebrae of the sacrum and the 4 fused vertebrae of the coccyx do not have intervertebral discs. Between the coccyx and the sacrum we have the **sacrococcygeal symphysis** that may allow limited movement between the two.

Ligaments connect various parts of the vertebrae to each other.

The spinal cord originates in the area of brain called the **medulla oblongata** and extends down the spinal column. It carries signals to and from the body (the **autonomic nervous system**) and allows reflex action (not controlled by the brain). It contains 31 pairs of nerves which connect it to skin, muscles, limbs, chest, abdomen, all internal organs. The nerves carry sensory information to the cords about conditions within the body, convey motor information to muscles and the sense of touch from the skin. The autonomic nervous system comprises of the **parasympathetic system**, which coordinates activities of the body when at rest; and the **sympathetic system**, which coordinates activities of the body when we become frightened or threatened.

During growth the spinal cord does not continue to lengthen as the spine grows. By adulthood it extends to the first or second lumbar vertebra L1/L2.

The spinal cord is protected by three layers of connective tissue. Outer layer (**dura matter**), middle layer (**arachnoid matter**) and inner layer (**pia matter**). The terminal part of the spinal cord is called the **conus dedullaris**. The pia matter continues as an extension called the **filum terminale**.

Cerebrospinal fluid (CSF) is a clear fluid that is in and around the brain and in the central canal of the spinal cord. It is produced in the brain, circulated around the brain and spinal cord and reabsorbed. A sample of CSF may be taken from the spine, in the lumbar region, to test for meningitis. This procedure is called a **lumber puncture.** However, removal of CSF from the spinal column may cause severe headaches.

Cerebrospinal fluid has many functions:

- **Buoyancy**: CSF allows the brain to maintain its density without being impaired by its own weight, which would cut off blood supply to the lower sections of the brain and thus kill neurons.

- **Protection**: it protects the brain from injury when jolted or hit and helps to protect the spinal cord.

- **Chemical stability:** removes waste from the central nervous system (which includes the spinal column).

- **Prevention of brain ischemia** that is restriction of blood supply.

The spinal cord is cushioned between the back and the front of each vertebra by the **epidural space,** which contains connective tissue and blood vessels

Bruising/trauma of the spinal cord may cause loss of sensation, impaired motor function, abnormal sensations or temporary paralysis below the level of injury. Injury to the cervical area may cause respiratory problems.

Severing of the spinal cord will cause total paralysis below that area; body function will be affected. Will result in death if cord severed above C4.

The lower lumbar region is inherently weak. Bad posture, weak abdominal muscles can only compound the problem resulting in lower back pain. Working the abdominals, transverse abdominis, internal and external obliques together with working the erecter spinae will help to strengthen the lower back.

Spondylosis

This is the term given to osteoarthritis of the spinal vertebrae in a degenerative form, due to wear and tear and age. It also affects the intervertebral discs of the spine – wearing away of the discs. The condition can lead to bone growths (spurs) on the vertebrae, chronic pain (due to compression of the spinal nerves), headaches and disability.

There are three types of spondylosis: cervical spondylosis (affects the 7 cervical vertebrae), thoracic spondylosis (affects the 12 thoracic vertebrae) and lumbar (affects the 5 lumbar vertebrae). All can lead to weakness of the back and limbs. Weight may also play part in aggravating the condition, as a strong back is reliant on strong core muscles.

Symptoms might not surface until the age of 40. Some factors that might trigger the onset of the condition include: neck or back injury, herniated disc, **spinal stenosis** (narrowing of the spinal cavity.

The condition cannot be cured. But treatment could help reduce symptoms. Treatment can include medication, physical therapy, exercise or surgery.

Here are some exercise to help strengthen the core and back.

- Exercises for the back:
    - Lateral pull down.
    - Chin up.
    - Seated pulley row.
    - Back extension.

- o One arm row.
- o Bent over row.

- Exercises for the core:

  - o Crunch.
  - o Reverse crunch.
  - o Figure 4 crunch.
  - o 90-90 crunch.
  - o Side bend.
  - o Prone plank.
  - o Side plank.

The list below shows the basic movements of the spine (spinal articulations). Cervical vertebrae, the ones from the base of the skull to the shoulder, are able to flex (i.e. tilt the head forward), **extend, rotate** and cause **lateral flexion** of the head by the following muscles:

- Sternocleidomastoid: twists, tilts the head.
- Semispinalis capitis: extends the head and flexes from side to side.
- Splenius cervicis: twists head.

Exercise to strengthen the lower spine include:

- Side lateral bend.
- Hyperextension.
- Core strengthening exercises.
- Exercises to strengthen the gluteals.
- Rotational exercises.
- Stretching exercises for the quads and hamstrings.

And finally when lifting free weights, you should always wear a belt because it helps to support the lower back and helps to maintain good form.

Chapter 27
Common injuries
And the R.I.C.E. Procedure

This section is all about common soft tissue injuries that we may experience from time to time, and what action to take following an injury. It also covers something called the R.I.C.E. Procedure. This procedure is simply four steps to take immediately after an injury occurs … which is rest, ice, compression and elevation.

R   Rest to prevent further damage to area.

I   Ice to help slow the build-up fluid around an injured joint, reduce blood loss from soft tissue to surrounding area, reduce pain.

C   Compression to reduce swelling, protection of area from further damage.

E   Elevation to reduce fluid accumulation around damaged area.

The three most common types of soft tissue injuries are **tendinitis, bursitis** and **bruise.**

- **Tendinitis** is inflammation of the outer surface of the tendon, caused by friction with adjacent bone.

  Treatment would be anti-inflammatory drugs. Use of the R.I.C.E. Procedure for the day or two after the onset of the condition. Ice should not be placed directly onto the skin. Use of bagged ice should be limited to about 15 minutes at a time, with long periods with the ice removed to allow the area to warm up again.

Exercises would include strengthening and stretching once pain has subsided and after a few days of rest.

- **Bursitis** is the condition where the bursae (sac of synovial fluid) becomes inflamed caused by increased friction with other structures, or sudden impact to the joint.

  An example would be bursitis of the shoulder after a sudden impact to the joint.

  Treatment would be the use of the R.I.C.E. Procedure. After which physiotherapy may be needed.

  Exercises to help ease the condition would be warming up and cooling down, stretching, strength training.

- **Bruise** (also called a contusion) is the condition where minor damage has occurred to skin, muscle resulting in trauma to blood vessels which leads to localised bleeding.

  Treatment may include the use of the RICE procedure, anti-inflammatory drugs.

  Exercise may be resumed after pain has subsided, but moderate at first to avoid further damage to area.

Sprain or Strain?

A sprain refers to the injury of ligaments cause by sudden wrenching movements. Whereas a strain refers to the injury of muscle or tendons. They can be classified in one of three ways:

- **First degree** is the least severe: minor stretching of tendons, muscles or ligaments. Might be mild pain, joint stiffness, and swelling. Not much loss of joint stability.

- **Second degree** is the result of some stretching, tearing of ligaments, muscles or tendons. Increased pain, swelling, and some loss of stability around the joint.

- **Third degree** is the result of complete tear or rupture of one or more of the muscle, tendons or ligaments. Severe pain, pronounced loss of stability, and major swelling is associated with this level of injury.

Overuse

Overuse is the term given to repeated exercise causing the muscles, ligaments and tendons to not have enough time to rest and repair before the next stress of exercise. Remember: rest your muscles more than you work them. Muscles only repair and grow during rest. Don't target the same muscles more than three times in one week. After working one set of muscles one day, give them at least two days of rest before working them again. In the days of rest for one group of muscles work a different group. The key is to not over do it!

Posture

Posture is the position and arrangement of your body and limbs. An example of bad posture in day to day habits would be slouching in a chair, which would put pressure on the lower lumbar region leading to back problems and pain. Good posture would be to sit up straight while seated. Strong core muscles would help to maintain good seating posture.

When referring to correct posture in a gym while using weights would mean not trying to move heaver weights than your capable of moving without contorting your body to help move the weights. Never try to exceed your boy's limitations. An example of bad posture, while using weights, would be when performing barbell curls ... swinging your body back and forth while curing the bar, instead of keeping your back straight, engaging your abdominals so your trunk remains stationary while you curl the bar.

What follows is a brief outline of the most common injuries that may occur.

A herniated disc

A herniated disc, also call a slipped disc or **prolapsed disc**, is one where the gelatinous core (known as the *nucleus pulposus* -- the spine's shock absorber) of the vertebral disc protrudes out through the fibrous outer coat of the disc to put pressure onto the spinal nerve. This could happen for a number of reasons: an accident, excessive pressure when lifting, wear and tear. Any disc in the spinal column can prolapse. However, the discs in the lower lumbar region are under more pressure because they have to support one's upper body and are reliant on a strong core and erector spinae muscles. Poor posture and/or bad lifting techniques and to a large extent excess weight increases the stresses already placed on the lower lumbar discs.

Symptoms of a herniated disc include: pain in back or neck, pain or tingling in the buttocks, back, legs, feet. Could also affect the control of bowel or bladder.

- Immediate treatment would be to rest, application of alternate ice and heat to affected area, anti-inflammatory drugs. None athletic activity for several days. Physiotherapy/massage may help to alleviate symptoms.

- Exercise to help you recover from a herniated disc would be those that target the spinal muscles and core muscles, like these:
  - Back extensions
  - Barbell roll-outs

- Stability ball curl up
- Back squat.
- Lateral pull downs
- Crunch
- Prone plank (targets the transverse abdominis. A deep muscle, lying under the obliques. It compresses the abdomen).

Frozen shoulder

Frozen shoulder, (**adhesive capsulitis),** refers to the limited movement of the arm around the shoulder. More specifically lack of full movement of the **humerus** (upper arm) around the **glenoid cavity** of the shoulder. This could be due to sudden impact to the joint, surgery, usage after prolonged immobility; and those who suffer from endocrine disorders (i.e. diabetes) have a high risk of developing the disorder.

The joint between the humerus and the **scapular** (shoulder blade) is called the **glenohumeral joint**. Four muscles called the rotator cuff support and stabilize the humerus. The **teres major** and **deltoid** also stabilize the joint. These six muscles are called the **scapulohumeral muscles**.

In the glenoid cavity there is a ring of cartilage called the **glenoid labrum**. Ligaments are attached from this to the head of the humerus.

Repeated tearing of the soft tissue around the joint results in scar tissue build up which restricts movement of the humerus. It is these adhesions of scare tissue that cause the loss of movement.

Symptoms include dull ache, or pain in shoulder, restricted movement. If left unattended the condition could get worse. Continued athletic use could result in further adhesion build up and eventually the need for surgical removal of scare tissue.

Rehabilitation would include moist heat and stretching to improve movements with approval from doctor and physiotherapist. Attempted full range of movements combined with strength training may help to avoid the onset of frozen shoulder. Before starting any exercise on the shoulder be sure to thoroughly warm all muscles, tendons and ligaments of the shoulder.

Rehabilitation exercise would include side lateral raise, upright row, and flat bench press.

Achilles Rupture

Achilles rupture occurs when the tendons from the **gastrocnemius** and **soleus**, the two calf muscles and the **plantaris** muscle are put such abnormal stress that the tendon tears. The Achilles tendon is the strongest tendon in the body. It has to withstand 3 to 12 times normal body weight when at rest.

Running, jumping etc. puts tremendous strain on the tendon, and if it is weak could tear. Sudden directional movements like in squash or hard acceleration could cause a rupture. The tendon inserts on the **calcaneus** (the heel bone).

Warming up, mild stretching and strength training will help to minimise the risk of Achilles rupture.

Rehabilitation of Achilles rupture would be to immobilise the leg to allow the tear time to repair. After which mild stretching and calf raises, squats would help to strengthen the muscles and tendon.

If Achilles strain is suspected in the gym then the use of RICE, anti-inflammatory drugs, followed by heat and massage to promote blood flow to the area and healing. A complete tear would see the need for immediate medical attention.

Patella ligament rupture

This is the tearing of one or more of the ligaments that are in and around the joint of the knee.

The tendon from the **quadriceps** muscles encapsulates and connects to the **patella** (knee cap) and the **prepatella bursa**. Then inserts on the tibia.

Anterior cruciate and **posterior cruciate** are internal ligaments that connect the **femur** to the **tibia**.

Fibular collateral ligament connects the **femur** to the **fibular**.

Tibial collateral ligament connects the **femur to the tibia.**

Rehabilitation for these ligament sprains, after a suitable rest period, would be static cycles, knee extensions, knee flexion, calf raises, static stretching, squat, and barbell step up. Duration and intensity of exercise should be built up slowly, increasing stamina and strength.

If injury occurred in the gym then the use of RICE if pain is not sever. If sprain is suspected then immediate medical attention would be required.

Shin splints

Shin splints or **medial tibial pain syndrome** or **periostitis** is the term given to pain experienced in the frontal region of the tibia caused be inflammation of the periosteum, a fibrous vascular membrane that covers bones. This could be caused by irritation of the tendons in that area, over use of the tibialis anterior (example would be running without proper conditioning and inadequate rest.

RICE would be used after the initial onset of shin splints. Then heat and massage to promote blood flow and healing.

Rehabilitation would include swimming, static cycling, leg extension, leg flexion. Apply heat before exercising along with static and dynamic stretching.

Hamstring strain

When **hamstring muscles** become stretched or torn this is called hamstring strain. The hamstring muscles are called **semitendinosus**, **semimembranosus** and **biceps femoris**.

This could be caused by a number of reasons: imbalance in muscle strength (quadriceps being much stronger than the ham strings), sudden explosive sprinting without proper conditioning. An untreated strain my lead to a complete tear.

Rehabilitation: heat before stretching and workout, which would include strengthening all the muscles of the leg. If you've a suspected hamstring strain but wish to run with the condition, then gradually increase the distance run while at the same time make sure symptoms do not become worse. Use resistance training to improve strength. However, rest more than you exercise, as a complete tear would need time to heal before undertaking any activity.

If a mild strain was suspected in the gym then use of RIICE procedure would be used to reduce the pain and swelling. Immediate medical attention would be required if a tear was suspected.

Tennis elbow and golfer's elbow

Tennis elbow (**lateral epicondylitis**) and golfer's elbow (**medial epicondylitis**) occurs when there has been repeated stress or sudden impact to the extensor muscle (tennis elbow), or the flexor muscle (golfer's elbow) of the forearm. In tennis elbow the lateral epicondyle becomes inflamed causing pain and restricted movement; in golfer's elbow it's the medial epicondyle which becomes inflamed with pain and lack of movement. The affected area of both is tender to the touch.

Rehabilitation for tennis elbow includes: biceps curl, chin ups, behind the neck pull down, press ups, dips. And for golfer's elbow behind the neck pull down, triceps extension.

If pain in the elbow joint is experienced while in the gym the use of RICE and rest for 2 to 3 days before attempting rehabilitation exercises.

House maid's knee

House maid's knee is the inflammation (bursitis) of the prepatella bursa (fluid filled sac in front of the kneecap). This could be caused by sudden trauma to the area or repeated pressure to the area (when kneeling); or an infection of the bursa.

If the bursitis of the patellar bursa is not due to infection then RICE and anti-inflammatory medication. Strengthening the muscles around the knee may help together with static and dynamic stretching after warming up. As well as keeping pressure on the bursa to a minimum.

If infection is deemed to be the cause then medical treatment would be required before attempting rehabilitation.

Lower back strain

This is the stretching or tearing of muscles or tendons in the lower back (in the lumbar vertebrae area). It can result from sudden trauma to the back, lifting incorrectly, sudden movement, making the muscles work too hard.

Rehabilitation exercises would include back extension, back squat, **erector stretch**, total back conditioning, including: chin ups, seated pulley rows. Plus exercises to strengthen the core muscles – **rectus abdominis, internal** and **external oblique, and transversus abdominis.**

If lower back strain is suspected while in the gym then rest on a firm surface on your back. Ice maybe used to reduce pain and swelling. Then heat to help mobility.

Muscle cramp

Muscle cramp refers to random firing of muscle fibres. This could be caused by one or more of the following: dehydration, the muscles being over worked, loss of **electrolytes** due to prolonged exercise (example would be sweating when running long distances). Sometimes sudden impact to the muscle may cause muscle cramp.

Muscle flexibility

Muscle flexibility refers to the range of movement of a limb. To become more flexible muscles, ligaments and tendons need to be stretched. This flexibility diminishes with age so it is vital to work muscles and to stretch as we get older.

Muscle hypertrophy

This is the term give to muscle growth due to tearing and repair of muscle fibres. This is what happens when we use weights to work our muscles with the goal of making them bigger.

When we start to exercise a muscle there is first an increase in the nerve impulses that cause muscle contraction. This alone often results in strength gains without any noticeable change in muscle size.

As the muscle is worked and rested it is natural for the muscle area to feel sore. This is normal – no pain no gain as the saying goes! This is because to make a muscle grow you need to create tiny tears in it. Muscle growth is the repair of these tears. This is the time when the muscle is adapting to the stress (increase in weight) that we have placed upon it.

As we continue to exercise, there is a complex interaction of nervous system responses that results in an increase in protein synthesis over months and the muscle cells begin to grow larger and stronger.

Don't over wok muscles as they grow when you are resting. Plan to have several days of rest between workouts.

Muscle fatigue

This refers to the muscle's inability to perform its normal working within normal parameters, like load etc. This could be due to over use, or lack of glucose, calcium, electrolytes. Remember rest more than you work out.

Chapter 28
The three body types

There are three body types. They are:

1. **Endomorphs.**

   This body type is characterized by wide hips, slow metabolism, soft and flabby body, bigger waist, round face and a high number of fat cells.

2. **Mesomorphs.**

   Characterized by an athletic build with a small waist, wide shoulders, low body fat percentage, and increased metabolism.

3. **Ectomorphs**

   Ectomorphs have a very thin frame, linear in appearance with small muscles, ultra-fast metabolism, low body fat, narrow shoulders, hips and waist.

Chapter 29

A very brief outline of Muscle structure

There are three types of muscle in your body:

- **Skeletal** … there are about 640 skeletal muscles in your body.

- **Smooth** … found in places like the stomach, intestines.

- **Cardiac** … only found in the heart.

Skeletal muscles have three main functions: motion, heat production and posture. Of these motion is the one function that people most associate with skeletal muscle. Heat production is a by-product of muscle activity. We take for granted the ability to position our body and limbs into a posture which we feel is comfortable; and even sitting in a chair we are using our strong back muscles to support our thorax so that we might be able to sit straight up. Our bodies are dependent on the functions of muscles. From raising our eyebrows to chewing food, transporting that food to the stomach; every breath we take; every movement that we make could not be achieved without muscles. The beating of our heart muscle gives us life.

Smooth muscle is under involuntary contraction, it is controlled by the autonomic nervous system. It is made up of bundles of long cells, each having a single nucleus. The intestine has a circular inner layer which contract to squeeze the intestine, and an outer longitudinal layer of muscle which produces wave like motion so as to move the contents of the intestine through it.

Cardiac muscle has cells which branch and interweave, they are Y shaped, have many nuclei, are shorter and wider than skeletal muscles cells, and which form bands around the ventricles of the heart. Cardiac muscle is controlled by the autonomous nervous system and the heart's pace-maker.

Let's now focus on the skeletal muscle. Here's a quick and simple overview.

A single skeletal muscle is in fact composed of thousands of muscle cells (**muscle fibres**). Down the length of each fibre are many sarcomeres. A **sarcomere** is the basic unit of contraction, and contains the contractile proteins (myofilaments) **actin** and **myosin**. Something called the Z band joins sarcomeres end to end. Each fibre is enclosed by a protective membrane called **endomysium**. Numerous fibres are bundled together into **fascicles**, which are covered by a layer of collagenous tissue called **perimysium**. These fascicles are grouped into a unit – the muscle we can see – which is encapsulated by **epimysium** tissue. These muscles are voluntarily controlled.

Each muscle cell or fibre needs huge amount of oxygen, fuel and calcium to work. Around the fibre is something called the sarcoplasmic reticulum which stores calcium. Throughout the entire muscle there is a network nerves, arteries and veins.

Contraction is the result of myosin attaching to actin and pulling. But this can only happen when calcium is released and attaches to actin which then rotates to expose binding sites that myosin can attach to. Only myosin that are ready to attach (those that have broken down ATP into ADP plus a phosphate) are able to attach to the binding sites. Once they have bound and pulled they let go of the ADP and the phosphate and are now ready to receive an ATP molecule. One ATP has attached the myosin binding head releases from actin and relaxes again. ATP that has attached to it breaks down into ADP and phosphate once more, ready for action again. The stored calcium is released when triggered by the nervous system. Muscle contraction is regulated by the proteins **troponin** and **tropomyosin.**

The muscle body becomes thinner at the ends and connects to tendons which then attach to bone. One bone is called the **origin** (the fixed bone) and the other is the **insertion** (the bone which the muscle moves).

Myoglobin is a protein found in muscle fibres of animals. It's there to store oxygen, and give oxygen to muscle fibre when needed.

Not all muscle fibres contract at the same speed. Some contract slowly – slow twitch; and some contract quickly – fast twitch.

Slow twitch or **slow oxidative fibres** contain large amounts of myoglobin, many mitochondria and many blood capillaries; these are called **type I fibres**. They split ATP at a slow rate, have a slow contraction velocity and are very resistant to fatigue and have a high capacity to generate ATP by oxidative metabolic process. Such fibres are found in large numbers in the neck, back and leg.

Fast twitch or **fast oxidative fibres** are of 2 types: Type II A and Type II B. Type II A contain very large amounts of myoglobin, very many mitochondria and many blood capillaries. They have a very high capacity for generating ATP by oxidative metabolic process, split ATP at a very rapid rate, have a fast contraction velocity and are resistant to fatigue. These are very rarely found in humans. Type II B are also called fast twitch or fast glycolytic fibres, contain a low content of myoglobin, relatively few mitochondria, relatively few blood capillaries and large amounts of glycogen. Type II B fibres are white, geared to generate ATP by anaerobic metabolic processes, not able to supply skeletal muscle fibres continuously with sufficient ATP, fatigue easily, split ATP at a fast rate and have a fast contraction velocity. Such fibres are found in large numbers in the muscles of the arms.

The fast twitch, type II a, moves 5 times faster than the slow muscle; and the super-fast, type II b, moves 10 times faster than the slow muscle fibre.

The average person has approximately 60% fast muscle fibre and 40% slow twitch muscle fibre. There can be variation in fibre composition, but essentially we all have three types of muscle fibre that need to be trained.

When talking about muscle growth, we are in fact talking about tearing muscle cells, and then resting so as the cells may have time to prepare. For this to happen protein is needed – more than is normally ingested; but not too much because as we know any that can't be used immediately is turned into fat. And don't forget, fat cells don't turn into muscle cells! This muscle growth is termed **muscle hypertrophy.**

And finally, **muscle atrophy** is the term given to the wasting away of muscle cells. This leads to weakness of the muscle. This could be due to disuse, nerve problems, injury, old age, improper diet, malnutrition, injury or disease of the nervous system.

Chapter 30

In which we have a few examples of skeletal Muscles and their function

We've all heard of the **calf** muscles, but how do they work? There are two separate muscles. One is called the **gastrocnemius** and the other is called the **soleus**. They perform relatively the same function, and that is to elevate the heel. The soleus works in a different position to the gastrocnemius, and that being with the knee bent. The soleus has its origins on the **tibia** (shin bone, upper posterior) and **fibular** (calf bone, upper posterior); its insertion is on the **calcaneus** (heal bone). Gastrocnemius has its origin on the **femur** (thigh bone), and its insertion is the calcaneus.

The **buttocks**, or **gluteals**, steadies the femur during standing. Each gluteal has three muscles. The lower part of the muscle also acts as an adductor and external rotator of the limb. **Gluteus maximus**, the largest muscle of the three, has its origins on the **Ilium** – the broad, large bone on the upper part of the pelvis. Its origins are on the **iliac crest**, **sacrum** (posterior) and **fascia** (connective tissue between groups of muscles and under the skin) of the **lumbar** (lower spine) area. It has its insertion on the femur and tibia.

The **quadriceps** – a group of four muscles – as a whole is to extend the knee. They are called the **rectus femoris,** which also acts a hip flexor because it crosses the knee; the **vastus lateralis, vastus medialis, vastus intermedius**. Origin is the Ilium and femur. Insertion is on the tibia.

The **hamstrings** – three muscles at the back of the leg – is to bend the knee they opposite to the quadriceps. They are the **biceps femoris, semitendinosus** and **semimembranosus**.

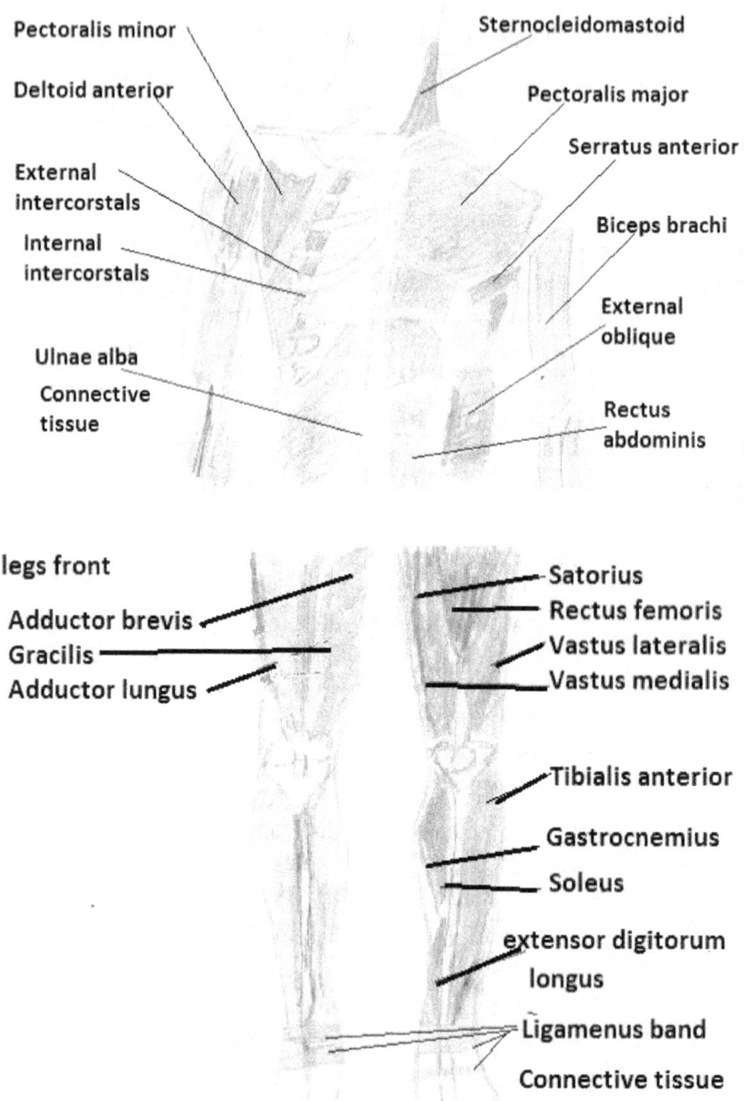
Front muscles
chest and arms
Pectoralis minor
Deltoid anterior
External
intercorstals
Internal
intercorstals
Ulnae alba
Connective
tissue
Sternocleidomastoid
Pectoralis major
Serratus anterior
Biceps brachi
External
oblique
Rectus
abdominis
legs front
Adductor brevis
Gracilis
Adductor lungus
Satorius
Rectus femoris
Vastus lateralis
Vastus medialis
Tibialis anterior
Gastrocnemius
Soleus
extensor digitorum
longus
Ligamenus band
Connective tissue

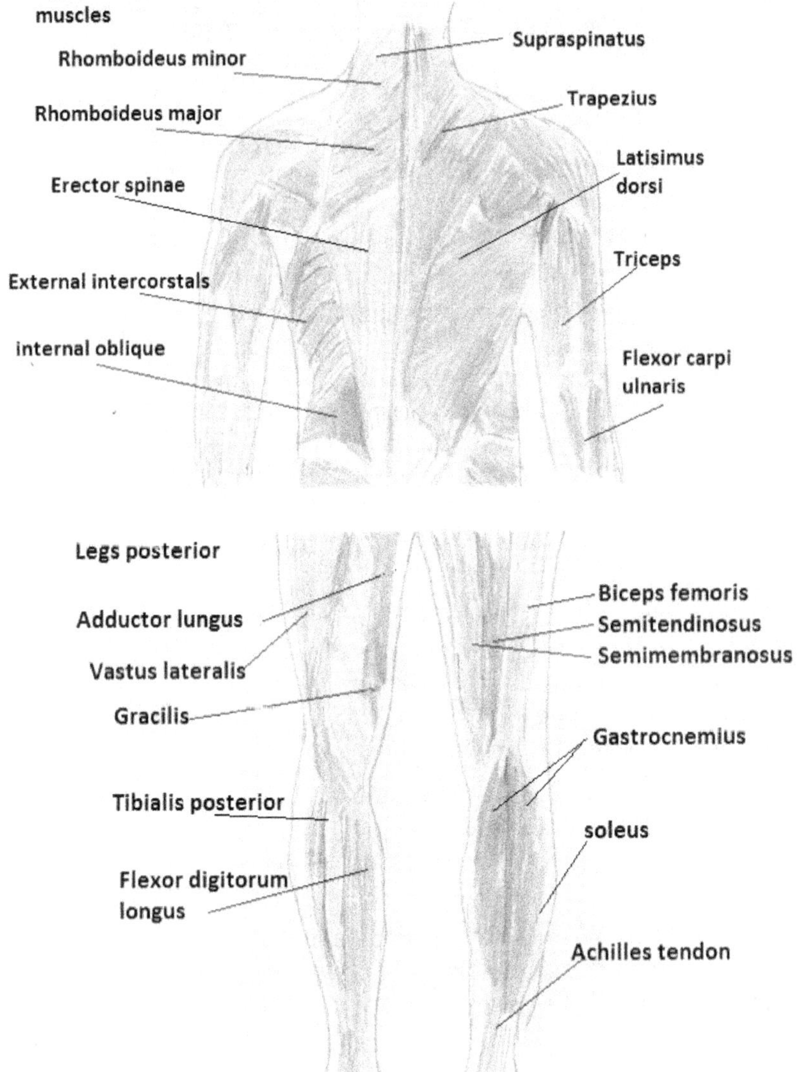

Upper body back and arm muscles
Rhomboideus minor
Rhomboideus major
Erector spinae
External intercorstals
internal oblique
Supraspinatus
Trapezius
Latisimus dorsi
Triceps
Flexor carpi ulnaris
Legs posterior
Adductor lungus
Vastus lateralis
Gracilis
Tibialis posterior
Flexor digitorum longus
Biceps femoris
Semitendinosus
Semimembranosus
Gastrocnemius
soleus
Achilles tendon

The **Trapezius** has many functions and these include scapular elevation (shrugging up), **scapular adduction** (drawing the shoulder blades together), and **scapular depression** (pulling the shoulder blades down). For the lower fibres of the trapezius, the origin is the spine and the insertion is the scapular; for the middle fibres the origin and insertion is the same as the lower fibres; for the upper fibres the origin is skull and the insertion is the clavicle.

The **hip flexors** are a group of muscles which pass through the pelvis that act to flex the femur that is to pull the femur towards the abdomen. The **adductor longus, adductor brevis** and **gracilis** are part of the hip flexor group.

The **deltoid** muscles essentially moves the arm away from the body: the anterior – front deltoid – raises it away to the front; the lateral deltoid – middle – moves the arm up and away to the side; and the posterior deltoid moves the arm away to the rear. Origin of the anterior muscle is the clavicle and the insertion is the humerus. For the lateral head of the muscle the origin is the scapular and insertion is the humerus. And for the rear muscle head the origin is the scapular and its insertion is humerus.

The **biceps** has 2 functions: its primary one is to flex the elbow (to move the forearm towards the shoulder); the second one is to **supinate** the forearm (turning the hand form a palms down position to a palms up position). Its origin is the scapular and its insertion is the radius.

The **pectoralis major and minor** bring the **humerus** (upper arm) across the chest. It also moves the shoulder area forward. Its origin is the clavicle and its insertion is the humerus.

The **Triceps** primary function is to extend the elbow (straighten the arm). Its secondary function is to bring the arm downwards. Its origin is the scapular and its insertion is the ulna.

The **erector spinae** group of muscles support the spine and extend it. They have their origin in the sacrum, ribs, lumbar, thoracic and cervical vertebrae. Their insertion points are ribs, cervical and thoracic vertebrae and the skull.

The **transversus abdominis** muscle is essential for trunk stability as well as keeping your waist tight. It has its origin at the lower ribs, iliac crest. And its insertion at the pubis, **linea alba** – connective tissue that runs down the middle of the abdomen.

The **obliques**, internal and external, work to rotate the torso and to stabilize the abdomen. The origins of the external obliques are the lower ribs; its insertion is the iliac crest. The origin of the internal obliques is the iliac crest; its insertion is the linea alba and part of the pubic bone.

The **rectus abdominis** muscle flexes the spine – to bring the rib cage closer to the hip. It has its origin at the pubis. And insertion at the 5th, 6th, 7th ribs and **xipoid process** – the lower part of the breast bone (**sternum**).

Latissimus dorsi – or **lats** – allows the body to bend from side to side; and pulls the arms down. Its origin is in the lower part of the spinal column. Its insertion is the humerus.

Serratus anterior stretches and rotates the shoulder blade. Works as an agonist to the rhomboids. Origin: ribs. Insertion: scapular.

Supraspinatus elevates the arm. Origin: scapular. Insertion: humerus (upper arm).

Flexor carpi ulnaris pulls wrist to the body. Origin: ulna. Insertion: fifth metacarpal bone in the hand.

Flexor digitorum longus helps to elevate the foot and stretches the toes.

Tibialis posterior moves the foot forward.

Tibialis anterior turns the foot up and inward; and also when walking is used to support the arch of the foot.

Here is a short list of general exercises – just a sample for each – for some of your skeletal muscles:

- **Biceps**

  Curl with free weights or machine weights. Incline dumbbell curl, concentration curl.

- **Triceps**

  Bench press with a close grip with free weights, overhead triceps extension, cable triceps push down, dumbbell kick back.

- **Calves**

  Barbell standing calf raises, Smith machine standing calf raise.

- **Chest**

  Bench press with barbell, dumbbell flys, cable cross crossover.

- **Forearms**

  Wrist extension and wrist flexion with a barbell.

- **Buttocks** (mainly gluteus maximus)

  Dumbbell or barbell squat or lunges.

- **Abdominals**

  Sit-up, abdominal crunch, figure four crunch, ball crunch, reverse crunch, v-leg raise.

- **External obliques**

  Wood chop (rotational movement).

- **Quadriceps** (cycling requires strong quads)

  Dumbbell spit squat, back squat, forward lunge.

- **Deltoids**

  Lateral dumbbell raise, front raise, rear lateral raise.

- **Trapezius**

  Barbell upright row, seated pulley row – at the end of the movement.

- **Erector spinae**

  Back extension.

- **Latissimus dorsi**

  Seated pulley row, chin ups, one arm row.

Chapter 31
Benefits of exercise

From the moment we embark on the road of physical training our bodies learn to adapt to the change we place on it. From being able to run that extra mile, bench pressing that few extra pounds, utilizing more oxygen, breaking down fat for fuel during moderate aerobic exercise, strengthening muscles around joints, encouraging bone formation with weight bearing exercise, our range of movements becoming greater as we gradually push our ability to stretch as in high kicks or splits. To memorize new movements and become faster in performing those movements in martial arts. Coordination, timing, power and balance are improved. Our confidence grows stronger as our bodies change and develop, take on a more muscular, athletic form, loose that lingering pound or two. Our BMI becomes lower or our body fat percentage drops another point. Our lungs become stronger, more efficient, our heart muscle become stronger – lowing our resting heart rate; our lymphatic system becomes more efficient – it relies on muscles activity to function properly; our skin becomes more healthy due to the fact our pores open during exercise which removes dirt and impurities; exercise stimulates intestinal movements resulting in more efficient waste removal; reduces blood pressure and thus reduces the chance of having a stroke; cartilage health in joints is maintained; more muscle means a higher metabolic rate to maintain the muscle; our joints remain healthier for longer so we are able to maintain our mobility and independence – everyday tasks like lifting the washing basket or picking up our children, releases endorphins which is the feel good hormone so stress is reduced; playing five a-side football or playing golf becomes less of a stress to our bodies as we become stronger and fitter.

Exercise. It's just one word but it has many beneficial factors for all of us as we get older. Take running for example. I for one love to run. I find it helps me to relax, concentrate, and solve problems. And these being just the side effects, for the real befits are to my body. Most of the time during my runs I run at a moderate pace where I'm using oxygen to burn fuel, but it's just below the point where my body would switch from aerobic to anaerobic – just that slight increase in pace and I stop breathing for a while as I pick up the pace and accelerate to a sprint for about 10 seconds or so; and then back down to my normal pace. But both the steady pace and the sprint have their benefits. During aerobic exercise the body learns to burn fat for fuel, the heart and lungs, diaphragm, intercostal muscles are worked. You feel as though you could take on any challenge. More oxygen is delivered to every part of your body. Then there are the sprints. The joints in the hips, knees and feet are worked harder as are the hamstrings and quads and the muscles that moves the foot away from the leg (plantar flexion) and bringing the foot towards the leg (dorsiflexion). Tendons are stretched that little bit further. Swinging the arms back and forth would work the shoulder muscles; and while holding the lower arm in a set angle would work the biceps in isometric contraction. Stamina is improved. For me personally I was able to build my running up to 11 miles twice a week, in my early 40s, with several sprints during the run and complete the 11 miles in 1 hour 27 minutes. Your body learns to adapt to the demands placed on it.

Resistance training again has many benefits: it increases muscle strength, efficiency, increases speed of muscle contraction time, increases metabolic rate, alleviates back problems, increases muscle flexibility and agility, improves one's physical appearance, helps to manage arthritis, increases muscle density so encourages bone growth, and so helps to prevent osteoporosis.

Both cardiovascular and resistance training have other benefits. They both reduce blood pressure. Reduces cholesterol levels. Increases high density lipoprotein (HDL or good cholesterol) in the blood. Reduces the chances of getting coronary heart disease. Stimulate digestion. Both burn up and remove toxins from the body. Help to maintain cartilage health in joints. Increases blood flow to the brain. Increases brain functioning by increasing the amount of oxygen delivered to it. Endorphin levels are elevated which increase resistance to pain. Exercising enhances mood. Provides a source of pleasure and fun. Releases anger and negative emotions.

The immune system becomes more efficient as it relies on muscles activity to function properly. Exercising reduces the severity of asthma. Allows you to overcome injury and illness quickly. Can relieve tension headaches. If you smoke exercising can help to reduce the urge to smoke because the adrenaline rush from a workout can replace similar feelings from smoking tobacco. It helps to regulate hormones. Improves glycogen storage due to the fact that muscles store glycogen, so the more muscle mass you have the greater the amount of stored glycogen. It helps to prevent or manage type 2 diabetes. Helps insulin to work better thus lowering blood sugar. Exercise alleviates menstrual cramps. In later years of one's life exercise befits the joints enabling one to be independent for longer, as well as the social aspect of being with people on runs or in the gym. Meeting new people and enhancing the quality of your life.

Exercising during pregnancy will help the mum-to-be carry the weight gain and be more prepared for the labour and birth. It will also make it easier to get back into shape once baby is born. Exercising could also help to prevent gestational diabetes, sleep problems, mood swings, back ache and posture. But remember: always seek medical advice before starting any exercise.

Nutrient supply to the body is increased during exercise. It reduces the chance of developing colon cancer. Also it stimulates intestinal movements, resulting in better elimination of wastes.

Exercise alleviates boredom. Lessens worry and tension. Reduces stress by removing lactic acid from the blood. Reduces anxiety and/or pain because the tranquillizing effects of exercise lasts for several hours. Enhances mood. Energy levels are increased during and shortly after exercising.

During strenuous exercise glycogen is broken down in the muscles to produce energy, which also produces, as a by-product, lactic acid. This lactic acid build up in the muscles is slowly removed from muscle tissue into the blood and transported to the liver where it is converted back to glycogen.

When we reach the age of 30 our body functions start to slow down. But exercise as we get older will help to slow down the ageing process.

Chapter 32

Exercise in pregnancy

Before starting any exercising plan during pregnancy always <u>consult your doctor first</u>. Only when you've been given the all-clear can you start to exercise. Exercise during pregnancy will help you carry the weight gain, be more prepared for labour and birth. It will also make it easier to get back into shape once your baby is born. But stop at about week 30. Exercising could also help to prevent gestational diabetes, sleep problems, mood swings, back aches and posture.

You should always start by warming up (like slow walking) and stretching as this will reduce the chance of muscle strain. Hold each stretch for 10 to 20 seconds. Warming up period should be between 5 and 10 minutes.

Don't use heavy weights but use lighter ones with more repetitions. Do not attempt any exercises which may reduce the blood flow to the uterus or your brain. Example would be bench press. Do any chest, back, leg or shoulder lifts in a sitting position or at an incline.

Relaxin is a hormone produced during pregnancy which slows down collagen production and at the same time increases collagen breakdown, and so softens connective tissue. Its primary role is to make birth easier; but its downside is loosen all joints in the body, including ligaments connecting bones. Exercise will help to strengthen muscles and work ligaments.

The pelvic floor muscle is a broad band of ligaments, muscle and tissue. It stretches from the pubic bone to the base of your spine at the back. It can be compared to trampoline in that it can stretch in response to weight and bounce up again; but becomes weak if too much weight is placed on it.

It supports your bladder and bowel; gives you control over them. It also supports the uterus; and affects the virginal muscles. If your pelvic floor muscle is weak you may leak a little urine when you cough, sneeze or exercise. Working the pelvic floor muscle after baby is born will help to reduce this.

Your temperature rises during pregnancy because after ovulation the follicle which released the egg turns into a corpus luteum, which produces high amount of progesterone. Progesterone is vital for establishing and maintaining pregnancy; but is raises the basal body temperature by 0.4 to 0.6 degrees.

You should avoid exercise which places the head lower than the chest for a number of reasons:

- blood pressure could drop
- faint
- become unbalanced

Avoid exercises that stimulate the nipples because it could be painful and may also lead to them leaking.

Do not work the chest area post-natally as this might induce lactation. Would also stress the uterus, which needs time to heal and reduce in size – bleeding might occur. Avoid exercise for a minimum of 6 weeks. Only restart with the doctor's go-ahead.

During pregnancy calorie intake should be increased by about 15%, combined with fibre, with protein increased by 15% at least so that baby can grow healthily. Complex carbohydrate such as fruit, whole-grain starches, potatoes, pasta, rice, cereals, corns and legumes should be the main source of energy. Meals should be small and frequent, as the digestive system slows down. Overall each meal should have a low to moderate glycaemic index. Try to avoid lots of citrus fruits.

Before and during exercising you should drink plenty of water and something light and easily digestible, like a cereal bar.

Exercise for no longer than 30 minutes at a time each day.

You should be able to safely commence training after at least 6 weeks from the time baby is born; and after you have been given the all clear from your doctor.

Chapter 33

A selection of diet plans

We all different reasons for going on a diet. Be it for losing weight or to gain weight, train for a half marathon – or a full one, or to get fit for playing sports. It's all too easy to sit back and enjoy comfort foods; and it can be hard to change your mind set to eat healthily. Each and everyone of us has different tastes, we love certain foods and hate others types of foods; some people have an allergy to certain foods. Some people are vegan or vegetarian. For some diets plans are a way of life and for others it's something new.

I'm not a dietitian, so what follows are basic diet plans that I had to design and submit which were part of the NABBA course that I took. The plans were for people to put on muscle mass or to lose weight, or simply healthy eating, by using everyday foods and supplements. I have not included special diets for those with allergies. Some of the diets included special treats like chocolate or a glass wine, some include meal replacements, which contain carbohydrate, protein and fat with vitamins and minerals. For each I found the value of protein, fat and carbohydrate from different books and just mixed various foods to obtain approximately the right percentage of carbohydrates to fat to protein.

Each diet plan was to be over seven days, with a variation of food each day for breakfast, lunch dinner and snacks. Some were with workouts and some were not. I found that the best way to present this was to use a spreadsheet with a separate entry for each item in the meal; and link all the values to give a meal total and a daily total of protein fat and carbohydrate. It took a while but I got there.

There were seven diet plans in total in the course but I'm showing three here Just as a note: when working out the percentage of protein, fat and carbs to the total Kcal for a meal, you might notice a slight error … it sometimes doesn't add up to 100, this is due to rounding of values to 2 decimal places.

So here's the first one. Healthy eating plan for a male with the occasional treat or two. Who doesn't go to the gym? The total calories each day to be around 2500, with different vitamins and minerals. He doesn't have any special dietary requirements.

Day 1

Breakfast

3 Weetabix, 200ml skimmed milk, 100g banana.

Total protein 14.65g, total carbs 71.75g, total fat 1.5g.

In terms of Kcal: protein 58.6, carbs 269.06, fat 13.5.

Total 341.16 Kcal.

In terms of percentage of total Kcal: protein 17.18%, carbs 78.87%, fat 3.96%.

Mid-morning

2 slices of wholemeal bread toasted with 10g olive oil spread.

Total protein 8g, total carbs 30.2g, total fat 7.1g.

In terms of Kcal: protein 32, carbs 113.25, 63.9.

Total 209.15 Kcal.

In terms of percentage of total Kcal: protein 15.3%, carbs 54.15%, fat 30.55%.

Lunch

1 carton(200g) low fat soft cheese, 1 whole grain role, 10g olive oil spread, 3 small (scotch) pancakes (90g).

Total protein 38g, total carbs 64g, total fat 26g.

In terms of Kcal: protein 152, carbs 240, fat 234.

Total 626 Kcal.

In terms of percentage of total Kcal: protein 24.28%, carbs 38.34%, fat 37.38.

Mid afternoon

1 carton (150g) low fat fruit yoghurt, 100g strawberries canned in syrup, 100g Del Monte pears in natural juice, Special K peach and apricot bar.

Total protein 8.8g, total carbs 66.4, total fat 2.7g.

In terms of Kcal: protein 35.2, carbs 249, fat 24.3.

Total 308.5 Kcal.

In terms of percentage of total Kcal: protein 11.41%, carbs 80.71%, fat 7.88%.

Dinner

100g grilled white fish, 300g sweet potato, 85g carrots, 125g spinach, 100g Belgian Chocolate ice cream (Haagen Dazs).

Total protein 34.4g, total carbs117.4g, total fat 24.17.

In terms Kcal: protein 137.6, carbs 440.25, fat 217.53.

Total 795.38 Kcal.

In terms of percentage of total Kcal: protein 17.3%, carbs 55.35%, fat 27.35%.

Evening

60g muesli with 200ml skimmed milk.

Total protein 13g, total carbs 50g, total fat 5g.

In terms of Kcal: protein 52, carbs 187.5, fat 45.

Total 284.5 Kcal.

In terms of percentage of total: protein 18.28%, carbs 69.91%, fat 15.82%.

Totals for the day:

Kcal: 2564.69.

Protein 116.85g which is 467.4 Kcal or 18.22% of total Kcal.

Carbs 399.75g which is 1499.06 Kcal or 58.45% of total Kcal.

Fat 66.47g which is 598.23 Kcal or 23.33% of total Kcal.

Day 2

Breakfast

60g muesli, 200ml skimmed milk, 150g low fat yoghurt.

Total protein 19g, total carbs 77g, total fat 6g.

In terms of Kcal: protein 76, carbs 288.75, fat 54.

Total 418.75 Kcal.

In terms of percentage of total Kcal: protein 18.15%, carbs 68.96%, fat 12.90.

Mid morning

2 slices (80g) wholegrain toast, 10g olive oil spread, 100g banana, 2 poached eggs.

Total protein 20.2g, total carbs 57.88g, total fat18.06g.

In terms of Kcal: protein 80.8, carbs 217.05, fat 162.54.

Total 460.39 Kcal.

In terms of percentage of total Kcal: protein 17.55%, carbs 47.14, fat 35.30.

Lunch

225g baked potato, 125g mixed salad, 100g tuna in brine.

Total protein 34g, total carbs 73, total fat 1g.

In terms of Kcal: protein 136, carbs 273.75, fat 9.

Total 418.75 Kcal.

In terms of percentage of total Kcal: protein 12.34%, carbs 86.12%, fat 1.54%.

Mid afternoon

100g grapefruit (fresh), 100g strawberries, 1 orange.

Total protein 3.6g, total carbs 26.8g, total fat 0.2g.

In terms of Kcal: protein 14.4, carbs 100.5, fat 1.8.

Total 116.7 Kcal.

In terms of percentage of total Kcal: protein 12.34%, 86.16%, 1.54%.

Dinner

100g turkey breast (baked/grilled), 125g (uncooked weight) noodles, 85g cauliflower, 85g peas.

Total protein 40g, total carbs 113g, total fat 11g

In terms of Kcal: protein 160 Kcal, carbs 423.75 Kcal, fat 99.

Total 682.75 Kcal.

In terms of percentage of total Kcal: protein 23.43%, carbs 62.07%, fat 14.5%.

Evening

68g Mars Bar

Total protein 2.85g, total carbs 46.92g, total fat 11.83g.

In terms of Kcal: protein 11.4, carbs 175.95, fat 106.47.

Total 293.82 Kcal.

In terms of percentage of total Kcal: protein 3.88%, carbs 59.88%, fat 36.24%.

Totals for the day:

Total protein 119.65g, total carbs 194.6g, total fat 48.09g.

In terms of Kcal: protein 478.6 Kcal, carbs 1479.75 Kcal, fat 432.81 Kcal.

Total 2391.16 Kcal.

In terms of percentage of total Kcal: protein 20.02%, carbs 61.88, fat 18.1%.

The next one is for a young male who just stated going to the gym, and wants to gain muscle. So we are looking for high protein with low fat in the meals. He needs to take in about 10% more Kcal per day than he needs to maintain weight, with protein going up to between 25% to 30% of total Kcal. You may notice that for the post workout value for protein is quite high. This is just one day and for one meal. Over the course of one day it evens out. But as we know any protein that cannot be broken down for amino acids would be turned into fat. However he is training in the gym each day. But by using a spreadsheet it is possible, by tweaking entries, to be more accurate.

I'm only showing 1 day here.

Breakfast

4 Weetabix with 300ml skimmed milk, 1 pear.

Total Protein 18g, total carbs 74g, total fat 8g.

In terms of Kcal: protein 72 Kcal, carbs 277.5 Kcal, fat 72 Kcal.

Total 421.5 Kcal.

In terms of percentage of total Kcal: protein 17.08%, carbs 65.84%, fat 17.08%.

Mid-morning

1 serving (25g) whey protein with 200ml water, 1 banana, 100g pineapple canned in syrup.

Total protein 21g, total carbs 40.7g, total fat 2.9g.

In terms of Kcal: protein 84 Kcal, carbs 152.83 Kcal, fat 26.1 Kcal.

Total 262.73 Kcal.

In terms of percentage of total Kcal: protein 31.97%, carbs 58.09%, fat 9.93%.

Lunch

3 poached eggs, 2 slices of wholemeal toast, 1 carton low fat fruit yoghurt, 100g strawberries canned in syrup.

Total protein 31.03g, total carbs 74.72g, total fat 16g.

In terms of Kcal: protein 124.12 Kcal, carbs 280.2 Kcal, fat 144 Kcal.

Total 548.32 Kcal.

In terms of percentage of total Kcal: protein 22.64%, 51.10%, 26.26.

Mid afternoon

CNP Pro Bar XS (39g chocolate flavour), 2 slices wholemeal toast with 10g olive oil spread.

Total protein 38g, total carbs 48.4g, total fat 11.6g.

In terms of Kcal: protein 152 Kcal, carbs 181.5 Kcal, fat 104.4 Kcal.

Total 437.9 Kcal.

In terms of percentage of total Kcal: protein 34.71%, carbs 41.45%, fat 23.84%.

Workout

500ml juice with 500 ml water.

Total protein 3g, total carbs 44g, total fat 1g.

In terms of Kcal: protein 12 Kcal, carbs 165 Kcal, fat 9 Kcal.

Total 186 Kcal.

In terms of percentage of total Kcal: protein 6.45%, carbs 23.53%, fat 4.84%.

Post workout

1 serving (72g) Pro MR meal replacement with 500ml water.

Total protein 42g, total carbs 16g, total fat 3g.

In terms of Kcal: protein 168 Kcal, carbs 60 Kcal, fat 27 Kcal.

Total 255 Kcal.

In terms of percentage of total Kcal: protein 65.88%, carbs 23.53%, fat 10.59%.

Dinner

125 turkey breast (baked/grilled), 100g noodles, 85g green cabbage, 85cauliflour, 85g carrots, 1 apple.

Total protein 44.56g, total carbs 85.38g, fat 9.03g.

In terms of Kcal: 178 Kcal, carbs 320.18 Kcal, fat 14.02.

Total 579.69 Kcal.

In terms of percentage of total Kcal: protein 30.75%, carbs 55.23%, fat 14.02%.

Evening

150g low fat fruit yoghurt with 2 rice cakes.

Total protein 7g, total carbs 42g, total fat 1.5g.

In terms of Kcal: protein 28 Kcal, carbs 157.5 Kcal, fat 13.5 Kcal.

Total 199 Kcal.

In terms of percentage of total Kcal: protein 14.07%, carbs79.15%, fat 6.78%.

Totals for the day:

Protein 204.59g, carbs 425.2g, fat 53.03g.

In terms of Kcal: protein 818.36 Kcal, carbs 1594.5 Kcal, fat 477.27 Kcal.

Total 2890.13 Kcal.

In terms of percentage of total Kcal: protein 28.32%, carbs 55.17%, fat 16.51%.

The next one shows the diet plan for one day for a female needing to lose weight. She likes chocolate and enjoys a glass of wine on an evening. Her daily Kcal is about 3000 calories. But for her diet cannot exceed 1200 calories per day. She does not go to the gym.

I'm only showing 1 day here.

Breakfast

1 slice wholemeal toast, 1 poached egg, 5g olive oil spread, 90ml orange juice.

Total protein 10.41g, total carbs 27.14, total fat 8.16g.

In terms of Kcal: protein 41.64 Kcal, carbs 101.78 Kcal, fat 73.44 Kcal.

Total 216.86 Kcal.

In terms of percentage of total Kcal: protein 19.20%, carbs 46.93%, 33.87%.

Mid-morning

2 finger KitKat.

Total protein 1.24g, total carbs 13.02g, total fat 5.48g.

In terms of Kcal: protein 4.96 Kcal, carbs 48.83 Kcal, fat 49.32 Kcal.

Total 103.11 Kcal.

In terms of percentage of total Kcal: protein 4.81%, carbs 47.35%, fat 47.83%.

Lunch

75g cottage cheese, 2 rice cakes.

Total protein 11.32g, total carbs 16.72g, total fat 3.94g.

In terms of Kcal: protein 45.28 Kcal, carbs 62.7 Kcal, fat 24.72 Kcal.

Total 143.44 Kcal.

In terms percentage of total Kcal: protein 31.57%, carbs 43.71%, fat 24.72%.

Mid afternoon

150g low fat fruit yoghurt, 1 pear.

Total protein 6g, total carbs 27g, total fat 7g.

In terms of Kcal: protein 24 Kcal, carbs 101.25 Kcal, fat 33.47 Kcal.

Total 188.25 Kcal.

In terms of percentage of total Kcal: 12.75%, carbs 53.87%, fat 33.47%.

Dinner

75g grilled chicken, 50g uncooked weight pasta, 125g spinach, 85g courgettes.

Total protein 31.78, total carbs 30.14g, total fat 4.07g.

In terms of Kcal: protein 127.12 Kcal, carbs 113.03 Kcal, fat 36.63 Kcal.

Total 276.78 Kcal.

In terms of percentage of total Kcal: protein 45.93%, 40.84%, fat 13.23%.

Evening

200ml glass of wine, 1 bar (26g) Miky Way.

Total protein 1.08g, Total carbs 19.84, total fat 3.67g.

In terms of Kcal: protein 4.32Kcal, carbs 74.4 Kcal, fat 33.03.

Total 111.75 Kcal.

In terms of percentage of total Kcal: protein 3.87%, carbs 66.58%, fat 29.56%.

Totals for the day:

Protein 61.83g, carbs 133.86g, 32.32g.

In terms of Kcal: protein 247.32 Kcal, carbs 501.98 Kcal, fat 290.88 Kcal.

Total 1040.88 Kcal.

In terms of percentage of total Kcal: protein 23.78%, carbs 48.26 Kcal, fat 27.96%.

So, there we have it! Just a few examples of simple diet plans. Maybe now you might go forth and design your own!

Chapter 34
Two examples of training schedules

What follows is a selection of exercise plans which I had to do for the course. There were various plans for general fitness, or to get fit to play golf, training schedules for the elderly, and so on.

One golden rule is to get the all clear from your doctor before starting training if you have any muscular or bone problems.

Before we go any further, let's take a look at the different types of muscle contraction relating to exercise:

- In **concentric contraction** a muscle contracts in order to lift a load which is less than the maximum that the muscle can move.

- In **eccentric contraction** the muscle resists lengthening. An example of this would be when once the biceps muscles have lifted a weight it needs to be lowered: the muscle while lengthening is also trying to contract.

- In **isometric contraction** the limb or body part that the muscle is trying to move remains static even though the actin filaments are moving across the myosin filaments. An example of this would be when one is trying to lift an immoveable object.

- In **isotonic contraction** occurs when the muscle shortens under a constant load. For example, when an object is lifted the muscle contracts and becomes shorter although the weight of the object remains constant.

Endurance training increases stamina and endurance. Exercises for endurance tend to be aerobic in nature. It develops slow twitch muscle fibres. Performing these exercises strengthens and elongate the muscles in preparation of extended periods of use.

Strength training comprises the use of resistance to muscular contraction to build strength and size of skeletal muscles. It can provide improvements in health and well-being including increased bone, muscle, tendon and ligament strength, improved joint function, improved cardiac function and increased bone density.

An **abductor** is any muscle used to pull a body part away from the midline of the body.

An **Adductor** is any muscle used to pull a body part towards the midline of the body.

All skeletal muscles work in pairs. As one muscle pulls the bone one way, the *agonist*, the other muscle, **antagonist**, relaxes.

Around most muscles **fixators** contract with no significant movement to maintain posture or fixate a joint. So they stabilize one part of the skeleton while another part moves.

For a small list of list of exercise reference books see the list of reference books at the back of this book.

And here we are, the first exercise plan. A young male with no ailment wanting general fineness. This is a twelve week program. He trains 4 times a week.

Session A

Weeks 1 – 6 Saturday and Tuesday – chest, back, arms.

Warm-up 10 mins either bike / cross trainer / row machine
Dynamic stretching 5 mins

Exercise	Sets	Reps
Dumbbell incline bench press	2-3	10-12
Dumbbell incline flys	2-3	10-12
Lateral pull downs	2-3	10-12
Dumbbell preacher curl	2-3	10-12
Triceps kickback	2-3	10-12
Upright row	2-3	10-12
Hammer curl	2-3	10-12
Ez barbell curl	2-3	10-12
Dips	2-3	2-4
Prone row	2-3	10-12
Dumbbell overhead press	2-3	10-12
Dumbbell flat bench press	2-3	10-12
Wrist extension	2-3	10-12
Wrist flexion	2-3	10-12
Back extension	2-3	10-12
Chin up	2-3	2-4
Internal rotation	2-3	10-12
External rotation	2-3	10-12
Dumbbell shoulder shrug	2-3	10-12

Cool down 5 mins: bike / cross trainer / walk.

Session B

Weeks 1 – 6 Sunday, Wednesday – legs, core, shoulders and cardiovascular.

Warm-up 10 mins: either bike / cross trainer / row machine.
Dynamic stretching 5 mins.

Exercise	Sets	Reps
Hip adductor	2-3	10-12
Hip abductor	2-3	10-12
Leg extension	2-3	10-12
Leg curl	2-3	10-12
Crunch	2-3	10-12
Figure 4 crunch	2-3	10-12
Reverse crunch	2-3	10-12
Back squat	2-3	10-12
Front raises	2-3	10-12
Side lateral raises	2-3	10-12
Bent over rows	2-3	10-12
Wood chop both sides	2-3	10-12
Run 10-12 mins 8 – 10 km/h	2-3	------
Plank hold 10 – 15 sec	2-3	-------
Side plank hold 10 – 15 sec both sides	2-3	-------
Calf raises	2-3	10-12

Cool down 5 mins bike / cross trainer / walk

Session A

Weeks 7 -- 12 Saturday and Tuesday -- chest back arms.

Warm-up 10 mins either bike / cross trainer / row machine.
Dynamic stretching 5 mins.

Exercise	Sets	Reps
Dumbbell incline bench press	3-4	6-8
Dumbbell incline flys	3-4	6-8
Triceps overhead extension	3-4	6-8
Dumbbell preacher curl	3-4	6-8
Triceps kickback	3-4	6-8
Upright row	3-4	6-8
Hammer curl	3-4	6-8
Ez barbell curl	3-4	6-8
Dips	3-4	6-10
Prone row	3-4	6-8
Dumbbell overhead press	3-4	6-8
Dumbbell flat bench press	3-4	6-8
Wrist extension	3-4	6-8
Wrist flexion	3-4	6-8
Back extension	3-4	6-8
Chin up	3-4	8-12

Internal rotation	3-4	6-8
External rotation	3-4	6-8
Dumbbell shoulder shrug	3-4	6-8

Cool down 5 mins bike / cross trainer / walk

Session B

Weeks 7 -- 12 Sunday Wednesday – legs core shoulders and cardiovascular

Warm-up 10 mins either bike / cross trainer / row machine.
Dynamic stretching 5 mins.

Exercise	Sets	Reps
Hip adductor	3-4	6-8
Hip abductor	3-4	6-8
Overhead split squat	3-4	6-8
Leg curl	3-4	6-8
Crunch	3-4	6-8
Figure 4 crunch	3-4	6-8
Reverse crunch	3-4	6-8
Back squat	3-4	6-8
Front raises	3-4	6-8
Side lateral raises	3-4	6-8
Bent over rows	3-4	6-8

Wood chop both sides	3-4	6-8
Run 12-15 mins 8 – 10 km/h	2-3	------
Plank hold 10 – 15 sec	3-4	-------
Side plank hold 10 – 15 sec both sides	3-4	-------
Calf raises	3-4	6-8

Cool down 5 mins bike / cross trainer / walk

And the second one is a twice weekly plan for legs, bum, tum with cardiovascular.

16 week program

Weeks 1 – 8

Warm up 10 mins either cross-trainer or static bike.

Dynamic stretching 5 mins.

Exercise twice weekly e.g. Monday and Thursday.

Exercise	Sets	Reps
Dumbbell step-up	2-3	10-15
Hip adductor	2-3	10-15
Leg curl	2-3	10-15
Leg extension	2-3	10-15
Fast walk / run 7- 10 mins each	2-3	-----
Crunch	2-3	10-15

Exercise	Sets	Reps
Reverse crunch	2-3	10-15
Side bend	2-3	10-15
Hip abductor	2-3	10-15
Row machine 5 mins each	2-3	-------
Barbell / dumbbell dead lift	2-3	10-15
Side bend – both sides	2-3	10-15

Cool down 5 mins bike / cross trainer / walk

Weeks 9-16

Warm up 10 mins either cross-trainer or static bike.
Dynamic stretching 5 mins.
Exercise twice weekly e.g. Monday and Thursday.

Exercise	**Sets**	**Reps**
Dumbbell step-up	2-3	10-15
Hip adductor	2-3	10-15
Leg curl	2-3	10-15
Leg extension	2-3	10-15
Fast walk / run 10-15 mins	1-2	-----
crunch	2-3	10-15
Reverse crunch	2-3	10-15
Side bend	2-3	10-15
Hip abductor	2-3	10_15
Cross trainer 10 mins	1-2	-------
Barbell / dumbbell dead lift	2-3	10-15

Side bend – both sides   2-3   10-15

Cool down 5 mins bike / cross trainer / walk.

Chapter 35
Supplements and what they do for you

Taking multivitamins and minerals supplements is a convenient way giving our body the daily intake of those that we need, for our body to function correctly and to stay healthy. Vegetarians and vegans my benefit from such supplements. Examples are calcium and iron.

Here is a list of common supplements.

- **Glucose**

  Could be taken by a diabetic before moderate exercise to avoid a hypoglycaemic attack.

- **Creatine**

  Could be taken to boost the skeletal muscle reserve of creatine and thus enhance muscle endurance and growth. The body produces about 3 grams of creatine per day which is stored in the muscles and used every time you work a muscle. A high dose of supplementation (20gram / day) should be avoided. A 3 gram supplement per day should not pose any health problems.

- **Gaba**

  It is a neurotransmitter, which means it helps nerve impulses cross the synapses. It also increases HGH (human Growth Hormone, which in turn helps to decrease body fat, promote an increase in lean muscle. It's believed to help relaxation and ease nervous tension.

- **Combination protein**

Is meal replacement. It contains a high amount for protein and carbohydrates together with some fat and dietary fibre etc., to be taken by those who wish to gain weight but find it hard, or do not have the time, to eat the high quantities of protein, carbohydrates etc. per day.

- **Evening Primrose Oil**

Said to relive eczema; and fight against rheumatoid arthritis; help premenstrual syndrome, menopausal symptoms; used for the conditions of cancer and diabetes.

- **Complex Carbohydrate Powder**

Replaces glycogen reserves during exercise.

- **Branch Chain Amino Acids**

Used for energy during exercise and can improve muscle recovery after exercise and build muscle growth.

- **Met Rx**

Brand name for a balanced meal replacement. Meal replacement products contains protein, carbohydrates etc. in a powder form which you mix with water or milk to provide a quick liquid meal before or after a workout. Could even be taken during a prolonged workout, which could be cycling, running or using weights.

- **Cod liver oil**

Has a high level of omega-3 and high levels of vitamins A and D. It is taken to ease the symptom of arthritis.

Pregnant women should not take cod liver oil supplement as it contains a high level of vitamin A. This is because studies have shown that taking cod liver oil during pregnancy could lead to child developing type 1 diabetes.

- **Omega 3 and 6 supplements**

  For diets lacking in these as they are essential to the body.

- **Star Flower oil**

  Has been said to have some benefits: helps alleviate eczema, may help to reduce the symptoms of rheumatoid arthritis.

- **Kelp**

  Is a seaweed. It contains mineral and trace elements, but in particular *iodine*, which is needed for the proper functioning of the thyroid gland.

- **Fat Burners**

  They work by increasing the body's metabolic rate, which in turn helps you to burn more calories.

- **Dandelion Root**

  Presumed to help with water retention.

- **Chromium picolinate**

  Said to prevent or treat chromium deficiency.

- **Whey Protein**

  Promotes muscle definition, recovery, repair and growth.

A list of reference books

Exercise

There are many books out there which show you different exercises either with machine weights or free weights that work the various skeletal muscles. Here are a few:

- The Men's Health Big Book of Exercise [ISBN 978-1-905744-69-5].

- Core Strength Training [ISBN 978-1-4093-4722-4] by Dorling Kindersley.

- Anatomy of Fitness Core [ISBN 978-1-7430-8007-8].

- Strength Training [ISBN 978-1-4053-4437-1] by Dorling Kindersley.

- Peak Physique [ISBN 978-4729-1257-2] by Hollis Lance Liebman.

Nutrition

- Nutrition a Health Promotion Approach [ISBN 978-0-340-93882-9].

- Sports Nutrition [ISBN 978-14081-0538-2] by Anita Bean.

- Calorie Counter [ISBN 978-0-00-731762-2] Collins Gem.

- Carb Counter [ISBN 0-00-717601-5] Collins Gem.

- Nutrition for life [ISBN 1-4053-0306-9] by Dorling Kindersley.

Human Body

- A pictorial Handbook of Anatomy and Physiology by Dr James Bevan [ISBN 1-85752-392-0].

- The Human Body [ISBN 978-1-8561-3007-3] by Dorling Kindersley.

- Molecular and Cell Biology For Dummies [ISBN 978-0-470-43066-8].

- Diabetes For Dummies [ISBN 0-7645-7019-6].

- The Anatomy of Sports Injuries [ISBN 978-1-905367-06-1].